A Workbook
of Practical
Skills

Psychiatric Occupational Therapy:
A Workbook of Practical Skills

**Peggy L. Denton,
M.S., O.T.R.**

*Occupational Therapy
Consultant,
Lake Geneva,
Wisconsin*

Little, Brown and Company
Boston/Toronto

Copyright © 1987 by Peggy L. Denton

First Edition

Fifth Printing

All rights reserved. No part of this book may be reproduced in any form or by any electronic or mechanical means, including information storage and retrieval systems, without permission in writing from the publisher, except by a reviewer who may quote brief passages in a review.

Library of Congress Catalog Card No. 86-80721

ISBN 0-316-18088-2

Printed in the United States of America

SEM

To my mother, who got me started;
To Bill, who helped me finish.

Preface ix

Contents

1. Effective Communication   1
   Getting Started 5
   Listening 12
   Responding 16
   Trying it Out 33

2. Assessment   41
   The Role of Theory 44
   Screening 51
   Evaluation 64
   Data Synthesis and Interpretation 88
   Trying it Out 99

3. Treatment Planning and Treatment Implementation   109
   Role of Theory 112
   Goals and Objectives 116
   Methods 128
   Implementing and Evaluating Treatment 148
   Trying it Out 156

4. Documentation   165
   Documentation 166
   Trying it Out 179
   Summary 184

Index 187

Several years ago, while teaching the psychosocial theory and treatment course in the occupational therapy program at the University of Wisconsin, I realized that the students needed a textbook of practical skills for psychiatric practice. Despite my best attempts to integrate theory with practice, students would almost inevitably ask, "But what do I *do* with the patient?" Neither students nor I were satisfied with the answer, "There isn't a cookbook." At the same time, drastic changes in the health care delivery system were limiting the time clinicians could spend training students in their fieldwork; thus, the students needed more advanced clinical skills in addition to theoretical knowledge, when they enter their fieldwork. It seemed that students could and should develop in school a minimum level of practical skills which would help them feel more confident, use their fieldwork more effectively, require less supervision from the clinicians, and, hopefully, increase their clinical competence. This book is an attempt to address that need.

My intent has been to write a transtheoretical workbook that strongly endorses using a theory base to guide the treatment process (assessment, treatment planning, and treatment implementation). Four occupational therapy frames of reference (functional performance, sensory integration, model of human occupation, and cognitive disabilities) are discussed and used to illustrate the treatment process. No attempt is made to discuss these in depth, and examples are given for comparison only. Further study of each of these frames of reference should precede or occur concurrently with using this book. Eliminating theoretical biases was more difficult than it first appeared, especially because I did not always recognize those that I had! I am grateful for Claudia Allen's thought-provoking review of my early work on this book; it jarred my thinking and stimulated my growth.

As every preface in every book states, no book is written alone, and this one is no exception. This book represents my professional development over the years, and so reflects the influence of the many patients, students, and therapists with whom I have been pleased and honored to work. It also represents the support and encouragement of many good friends. In particular, I am indebted to Bill Johonnott, who unfailingly and lovingly listened, critiqued, edited, prodded, and typed this book to its conclusion; to Susan Cunningham for her constant encouragement; and to Neal and Ginevra Ewers for their faithful support. Gratitude is also expressed to Karen Bonjour, Lisette Kautzman, Helene Archibald, and Carol Holmes for their perceptive and helpful feedback along the way. Barbara Ward, former allied-health editor of Little, Brown and Co., is also acknowledged for her continued faith that some day I would get this book done.

I presume that this workbook will be used in conjunction with level 1 or 2 field work. It includes many exercises for applying the concepts that are discussed. You will benefit most from this book if you do the exercises and discuss them with a colleague or fellow student. Answers are not included because the intent of the exercises is to stimulate your ability to solve problems and trust your own judgment. There are numerous places in which the limits of our empirical knowledge are pointed out. These are intended to provoke your thinking and stimulate you to contribute to the expanding knowledge base of psychiatric occupational therapy. Most of all, I hope that you find this workbook stimulating and enjoyable and that it contributes to your development of clinical skills.

P. L. D.

The problem with communication is the illusion that it has been accomplished.

George Bernard Shaw

On the first day of her fieldwork placement in psychiatry, Jo's supervisor suggested she start to work with Mr. Smithson. Jo felt excited. *Finally, a patient!* she thought. *After all that studying, I finally get to put some of it into practice.* "Hello, Mr. Smithson. My name is Jo Rabson," she started. "I'm a new occupational therapy student and I'll be working with you." Suddenly Jo was overwhelmed with anxiety. *What should I ask next?* she thought. *What should I do if he looks like he doesn't want to talk? How can I get across that I'm interested and concerned without looking like I'm insincere and phony? Will I know what to do if he starts to tell me anything important? Can I really understand enough about what he's going through to empathize? He's getting gypped, having a student working with him instead of a "real" therapist. Will I really be able to help? Usually, it's not hard for me to talk with people. Why is this so hard?*

This scenario represents a common struggle with beginning therapists. Although the desire to "work with people" and "be helpful to others" represents the major reason for choosing occupational therapy as a profession, meeting a patient for the first time can be inherently frightening [26]. Jo knows she is a good listener and often very helpful to her friends; then why should it seem that all of her communication skills vanish when she needs them most?

Reiser and Schroder suggest that most students experience three general anxieties at this stage of their training: (1) self-consciousness about his role*, (2) fears and fantasies about what constitutes professional behavior, and (3) uncertainty about how to proceed technically with patients [33].

Self-Consciousness

Students frequently report that they initially hesitate to "do too much" with the patient because "the patient deserves the benefit of a real occupational therapist, not just a student." This fear that your learning comes at the patient's expense can create doubts that the patient will want to work with you, a student. Although it may not always seem like it to you, you are a "real occupational therapist" (in training) and you are seen that way by your patients. The manner in which you handle this issue can assuage or enhance feelings of uncertainty for both you and your patient. Neither of you benefits by a self-disclosure of "Hello, my name is Jo. You're my first patient, and I don't know much about what I'm doing yet, but I'm anxious to learn." Conversely, false bravado does not help either you or your patient. An honest, sincere introduction of yourself and role (occupational therapy [OT] student, affiliate, or intern) usually suffices.

Public and legal recognition exists for practical training in our profession; thus, most licensure laws that regulate clinical practive provide for training students under qualified clinicians. As you probably know, you are operating under the licensure or certification of your supervisor. Even though you may be given primary responsibility for a patient, your supervisor assumes legal and professional responsibility for your work, including liability for negligent and inadequate treatment [45]. Communicating well with your supervisor is essential to your development as a responsible, skilled clinician.

Professional Behavior

From the day you were first introduced to the concept of therapeutic use of self in O.T. 101 (Introduction to Occupational Therapy) you were told that how you are with a patient is often as important as what you do with him. What does constitute

---

*To avoid the use of "him or her" and "he and she" throughout book, I have used the masculine or feminine personal pronoun to indicate therapist and patient. Such usage certainly does not indicate any gender bias. *P.L.D.*

professional behavior? You are advised to empathize but not sympathize, encourage rather than praise, care but not get overinvolved, and to be friendly but not a friend [12,21,31,40]. In addition you are encouraged to know yourself, be honest, genuine, and respectful, and aim to make your therapeutic relationships accepting, dynamic, purposeful, honest, realistic, and responsible [5,6]. Finally, be careful. "All helping is for better or worse. No helpee is left unchanged by any helping interaction . . ." [9]. At the same time, you are frequently advised not to discuss anything personal with patients, not to get "too close," and to leave your job at the office, not take it home with you. Although probably designed to save you the pain and sadness of overidentifying with a patient (an experience doubtlessly shared by almost all occupational therapists), these guidelines are confusing. How can you be friendly and genuine and not disclose anything about yourself? Suddenly your natural communication skills seem inappropriate. An excellent discussion of how effective therapists integrate personal and professional qualities can be found in Purtillo's *Health Professional/Patient Interaction* [31]. You are encouraged to think about these issues throughout the rest of this text, because your communication skills are directly related to your clinical effectiveness in assessment, treatment planning, and implementation. Rediscovering the therapeutic potential of one's own personality is one of the most important goals of any introductory experience [33].

Proceeding Technically
The rest of this chapter is designed to help you develop the communication skills for helping people into effective action. Communicating well involves attending, listening, and responding in a manner that facilitates your patient's self-exploration and growth. Being able to say what you think you said so that others think they know what you mean is not easy. Fortunately, there is evidence that communications skills can be learned [7,42,43]. Through self-evaluation, practice, feedback, and continued practice, these new skills become part of your style. Perhaps you feel you already are a good communicator: After all, it just takes common sense. Right?

Your Turn
Take a look at the following common sense responses, and check off any that you have said while trying to be helpful.*

_____ 1. You should have . . . You know better than . . .
_____ 2. Why don't you try . . . My advice is to . . . You'll feel better if . . .
_____ 3. If you think that's bad . . . When that happened to me, I . . .
_____ 4. The reason you feel like that is . . . What you need is to . . .
_____ 5. You have to . . . You must . . .
_____ 6. Why . . . Who . . . What . . . When . . . How . . . (in rapid succession)
_____ 7. Here's where you're wrong . . . The facts are . . . Yes, but . . .
_____ 8. Come on, it's not so bad . . . Don't feel that way . . . Don't worry . . .

Each of these common sense responses can evoke unintentional feelings in your listener. Look at them again. Think about how you would feel if you were trying to discuss a serious problem with a friend, and you heard the following responses. Describe your feelings in one or two words.

*Adapted from: J. N. Weismer Communication Effectiveness: Active Listening and Sending Feeling Messages. In J. W. Pfeiffer and J. E. Jones (eds.), *Annual Handbook for Group Facilitators*. La Jolla, CA: University Associates, 1978.

1. *Evaluation.* You should have . . . _____
2. *Bartender.* Why don't you try . . . _____
3. *Sore thumb.* If you think that's bad . . . _____
4. *Analyst.* The reason you feel like that is . . . _____
5. *Sergeant.* You have to . . . _____
6. *Crowbar.* Why? Who? What? When? How?_____
7. *Professor.* Here's where you're wrong . . . _____
8. *Devaluator.* Come on, it's not so bad . . . _____

Although these responses may be well meaning, they do not necessarily communicate that intent. Since you are in a caring profession, one can assume that you are genuinely interested in your patient's welfare and wish to communicate that interest. This chapter contains information and exercises that will help you through the first three steps of improving your communications skills—identifying effective skills, assessing your own performance, and practicing. You will gain the most if you are honest with yourself when assessing your own performance. The final two steps—seeking feedback and continuing practice—are up to you to do on your own. All five steps are necessary for complete and lasting growth.

One final note—throughout the chapter, you will find references to you as the therapist communicating with your patient. These terms are used only as reference points. There is nothing magical about these communication skills that make them "for therapeutic use only." Practice them in all of your relationships with your professors, clinical supervisors, team members, and friends and discover what happens!

"Would you tell me, please, which way I ought to go from here?"

"That depends a good deal on where you want to get to," said the Cat.

"I don't much care where—" said Alice.

"Then it doesn't matter which way you go," said the Cat.

"—so long as I get somewhere," Alice added as an explanation.

"Oh, you're sure to do that," said the Cat, "if you only walk long enough."

Lewis Carroll
Alice's Adventures in Wonderland

The first step in establishing a helping relationship is to get your patient fully involved. It might seem that if a person seeks help, he would naturally be invested in the treatment process. Unfortunately, this is not always the case. The drop out rate of psychiatric treatment is high; for instance, one study revealed that it was 40 percent after just one session [39]. To date no study has been done that indicates O.T. compliance in either inpatient or outpatient treatment settings, but there is no reason to assume that O.T. would be different from other professions. Failure to attend outpatient appointments and resistance to treatment are well-documented problems encountered by most psychiatric professionals.

Carkhuff and Anthony look at the helping relationship as an interconnected process in which the actions of the helper and helpee (therapist and patient in this case) are linked [9]. The actions taken by you, the therapist, can either facilitate or hinder the actions taken by your patient. You can help promote your patient's active involvement in O.T. by using preparing and attending actions.

Preparing

Preparing involves preparing the patient for your interaction (i.e. an interview, evaluation, or O.T. group) and preparing the setting in which you treat the patient.

Preparing the Patient

The initial contact with your patient is critical in creating an atmosphere of trust and concern. This is a good opportunity to start building rapport, but too often this contact is made haphazardly or hastily without thinking about the overall impression being made.

NONVERBAL

All communication has both a verbal message, or what is said, and a nonverbal message, or the way it is delivered. Very often the nonverbal message conflicts with the verbal content thus confusing the listener. Start by looking at the nonverbal impressions given by various methods of making the initial contact. The content of the message is discussed in the next section. For now, focus on how the message is delivered.

Your Turn

Which method(s) would you use to inform your patient that you would like him or her to come to O.T. this afternoon?

____ 1. Post a notice on the bulletin board by the nurses' station so he will be sure to see it.

_____ 2. Have the doctor announce O.T. time at the community meeting this morning and remind all people referred to O.T. to attend.

_____ 3. Introduce yourself to your patient, tell him about what you do in O.T., and ask him to come this afternoon.

_____ 4. Ask another patient you know who comes to O.T. to bring the new patient along with him.

_____ 5. Have the nurse or psychiatric worker find your patient 10 minutes before O.T. and ask him to attend.

Take a look at each of these methods again, and write about the nonverbal message conveyed with each one. Are there times when each one might be effective?

Method   _Impression_

1. Notice on bulletin board

2. Doctor announcement

3. Personal invitation

4. Invitation by another patient

5. Reminder by nurse or mental
   health professional

CONTENT

Next, pay attention to the content of your message. Because people often need help with motivation, you must explain in a manner that he can understand, what your patient will be doing in O.T. and what he will get out of it. For example, suppose one of your professors announced several additional required assignments for a class. Although you chose to attend college and have willingly expressed a desire to learn, you probably would not readily agree to these assignments unless you understood exactly what was expected of you and what you would gain from the extra work. Your patients are often in similar situations. Continually explaining the role of O.T. may seem tiring and frustrating to you, but it is inhereent in our profession. If you are ready with a well-thought-out explanation, you will be able to present yourself more confidently and convincingly.

Your Turn

In the space below, write an explanation of O.T. in psychiatry that would be appropriate to use with your patient. In other words, leave psychobabble buzzwords out!

Check your definition out by trying it out on a friend who is not an occupational therapist. If you get a blank or confused look, go back to the drawing board!

Preparing the Treatment Setting

Before your patient arrives, make sure the physical setting encourages his active participation. Carkhuff and Anthony describe the best physical arrangement for a one-to-one session as two chairs facing each other about three to four feet apart. An oval pattern of chairs for a group allows you to see everyone in the group without turning your back [9]. Tables provide barriers, but they can also provide a sense of security. Try to sit across the table corner from your patient so you have the smallest possible barrier between you and so you can see each other without having to turn. Even though this is ideal, do not rule out going for a walk or sitting side-by-side while working on a project as good opportunities to talk with your patient. (Remember the good heart-to-heart talks you had with your mom while doing dishes or with your dad as he drove you somewhere?) There are times, especially early in the relationship, when mutual involvement in a task that does not require sustained eye contact provides a safe environment in which your patient can talk comfortably with you.

Another aspect of the treatment setting to prepare is the atmosphere. What type of overall impression does the O.T. space give? Are materials organized for easy and logical use? Are the space and privacy adequate for the types of activities done in the room? How much stimulation do the space and materials provide? In general, occupational therapists consider the nature of the patient's environment and its effect on his performance as part of the treatment domain [3,13,23]. For example, the manner in which materials and activities are used with the patient is recognized as an important treatment variable in all O.T. theoretical frames of reference [1,4,10, 15,24,28,35]. However the overall organization of materials and supplies in the O.T. treatment environment is rarely noticed or discussed. Samples of work with prior patients can help stimulate curiosity and involvement. On the other hand, a messy area can give the impression that you are disorganized and too busy for the patient. You may have days when you feel that you could not give your job away since "no one would take it," but a wall poster expressing that does not present a positive helpful outlook. O.T. spaces, as a general rule, suffer from sensory overload. There are things stacked, posted, sitting, and hanging all around. Just as a person's home is a reflection of his personality, the O.T. space is a reflection of how you conduct your business. The amount of stimulation and the nonverbal messages about you, which the patient receives, can have a strong impact on his willingness or ability to get involved. Too little or too much arousal is experienced negatively as a loss of control or a lack of opportunity to exercise one's capacity to act [3].

Your Turn

Take an objective look around an O.T. space and notice the nonverbal impressions given. Are they helpful? In what way? Could there be improvements? State your reasons in the space below. Try to look at the area as though you had never been there before.

Attending

Your attending actions show your patient that you are interested in him and willing to help. Learning how to attend to a patient is important in many counseling approaches [9,14]. Ivey and Authier feel that adequate attending is so critical it is the core of their microcounseling approach [22]. Attending involves both verbal and nonverbal actions.

A story is told of a grade school teacher who started her class in the fall with her usual opening of "I'm so happy all of you are in my class and I'm sure we will have a very enjoyable year." One youngster raised his hand and said, "Mrs. Jones, if you are so happy to be here, you should tell your face!" Nonverbal messages may not outweigh verbal messages, but if they contradict the person's verbal message, the receiver feels confused. How would you interpret a low voice between clenched teeth hissing, "I am not angry!" Observing the degree of congruence between a person's verbal and nonverbal messages is an important clue to understanding the person better (see Listening, page 14). Likewise, being aware of your nonverbal messages and the congruence between your nonverbal and verbal messages helps to ensure that your message is received as you intend.

Positioning

The position of your body relative to your patient gives a strong nonverbal message. Carkhuff and Anthony suggest that you consider three aspects of your position: level, angle, and inclination [9]. Each gives a distinct nonverbal message.

Your Turn

Several common positioning arrangements follow. Write down the nonverbal message that you are giving with each one.

1. *Level.* The "professional perch" is sitting on the edge of your desk or standing while your patient sits.

   Nonverbal message:

2. *Angle.* Sitting turned slightly to the side without facing your patient directly.

   Nonverbal message:

3. *Inclination.* Leaning back in the comfortable, rocking swivel chair.

   Nonverbal message:

Certainly no one intentionally tries to put the patient in a subservient position, but busy therapists sometimes appear to fly reconnaissance around the perimeter of the group, swooping in to offer assistance by leaning over the patient's shoulder. You are giving a nonverbal message with the manner in which you position yourself with your patients. Monitor yourself so you are aware of what this message is.

Eye Contact

Making eye contact with your patient is critical to establishing rapport and developing a helping relationship. Of all the nonverbal behaviors, eye contact seems to be the one that is most strongly interpreted accoding to social and cultural norms. For instance, studies have shown that people were attributed a higher professional status if they made eye contact more while talking than while listening. Women appear to make eye contact more than men do, but this is highly variable according to situations. Culture also influences eye contact patterns [19,25]. Because eye contact is greatly influenced by attributed power, gender, and culture, your values about appropriate eye contact may not be the same as your patient's. You are probably familiar with the professional, practiced gaze in which the person seems to be looking at you but is actually focusing just about an inch to the side of your eyes or just over your shoulder. This gaze is worse than no eye contact, because it conveys a nonverbal message of disinterest and lack of involvement. Carkhuff and Anthony suggest that eye contact be frequent and maintained for at least 20 seconds [9]. Connecting with your patient through vision demonstrates your genuine and sincere interest in him.

Your Turn

Engage a person you do not know well in a discussion, and try to pay attention to your own eye contact patterns.

Did you maintain eye contact more when you talked or when you listened? _____
Was your eye contact related to your desire to be liked by the person to whom you were talking? _____
Was your eye contact affected by the gender of the person to whom you were talking? (Be honest!) _____
Was your eye contact affected when you did not agree with the person to whom you were talking?_____

Back Channels

Other attending actions such as "uh-huh," "ya," "um," nodding your head, or smiling can also demonstrate your interest. Use them carefully. The critical ingredient is not the action itself, but its timing and sequence. These encouragers, called back channels, usually come at the end of a long pause or when the patient turns his head towards you. Absence or unexpected placement of these back channels has been shown to cause the speaker to hesitate more, touch his body more (a measure of insecurity), or to stop talking [25]. This makes sense. You know how disconcerting it can be when you are in the middle of a serious story, and the person listening to you breaks out in a grin! Perhaps you have seen the novice counselor who has obviously been told that uh-huhs and nods are important, but lacks timing. Constant head bobbing and uh-huhhing give the impression that he is responding automatically and without interest.

Your Turn

Use a friend for this discussion, because you need someone who can give you honest feedback. Back channels are hard to detect on your own. Talk about a variety of topics including some about which you disagree. Assess your own use of back channels, and then ask for feedback.

Which of the back channels did you use most frequently?

Was your timing generally appropriate?

Did you find that any of the back channels seemed to encourage further discussion?

Did the topic of discussion affect either the type or amount of back channels?

Were there any differences in your self-assessment and the feedback from your friend about your back-channel use?

If so, how do you account for this difference?

Nurturing

Nurturing, or attending to the patient physically, is another way to show your interest and willingness to help. Purtillo suggests nurturing can occur in four ways [31].

1. *Personal hygiene.* Providing the basics such as a tissue, apron, or gloves when needed can turn your patient's embarrassment into comfort.
2. *Personal comfort.* Providing juice or water can alleviate your patient's dry mouth that often accompanies psychotropic medication.
3. *Personal interest.* Remembering a birthday, admiring a dress or shirt, talking about a special interest, and remembering and spelling the patient's name correctly are all ways that indicate your interest in him as an individual.
4. *Expanding awareness.* Getting the daily newspaper, bringing in seasonal flowers, or talking about a new movie can help remediate the disorientation and isolation that occurs so frequently in the hospital.

Mosey suggests that people have inherent universal health needs that are different from those needs that arise from pathology or inadequate psychosocial development. She suggests that addressing these health needs should be an essential, if not primary, emphasis of treatment in hospitals and community settings [11,27]. Nurturing your patient can meet some of his health needs while fostering the development of your relationship. Nurturing, however, is not a substitute for treatment, and it should not be confused with your need, at times, to provide direction and make therapeutic interventions. It is possible to be nurturing while still setting limits and encouraging your patient's independence. Effective use of self is discussed further in Chapter 3; however, for now, concentrate on the nurturing actions that demonstrate your genuine interest in your patient.

Your Turn

List 10 nurturing actions that you can use with your patient in your fieldwork setting. Try them out and note the results.

Action   *Result*

1. _____   _____
2. _____   _____
3. _____   _____
4. _____   _____

5. _____   _____

6. _____   _____

7. _____   _____

8. _____   _____

9. _____   _____

10. _____   _____

Summary

Helping your patient become fully involved is the first step in the treatment process. In this section, you have been introduced to specific preparing and attending actions that demonstrate your sincere interest and willingness to help. Both are important for this first step, but they should also permeate your entire relationship. They help your patient become and stay invested in the treatment process.

It's hard to hum a tune and contemplate your own death at the same time.

Woody Allen

Mother: I'd like you to take out the . . . , are you listening to me?
Child: Yes, Mom, I hear you.
Mother: Yes, but are you *listening* to me?

Sound familiar? Because we spend so much of our day listening, it makes sense that we should be very good at it; however, that doesn't seem to be the case. Carkhuff found that people remembered only about half of a short talk immediately after they heard it [8]. Because most people can comprehend speech three to four times faster than normal conversation, this poor rate of recall seems to be due not so much to a *lack of time* to listen, but *too much time.* The key to effective listening then is what you do with your extra listening time.

Listening Blocks

Effective listening is an active process in which the listener interacts with the speaker. Understanding what blocks effective listening is the first step in improving your own listening skill. Rogers suggests that most people neither listen openly nor evaluate constantly what they hear because they fear their attitudes may be influenced [34]. Effective listening can be blocked in several ways [37].

Thinking about the Person

Making judgments about a patient's lifestyle, morals, or manner of behavior and speculating on his motivation for his behavior severely limits your ability to hear and understand. Judgments become most problematic when the person, the topic of discussion, or both do not fit our personal value system. Hearing what the patient is saying from his perspective becomes difficult when strong feelings are aroused. Rogers designed an exercise to help train therapists to overcome this problem [5]. Two people are asked to discuss a topic about which they disagree. Each is allowed to say whatever he wishes, but, before voicing his own views, each is to restate the ideas and feelings expressed by the other participant to that person's satisfaction. If each person could repeat what the other person said and felt, then he heard and understood and was paying more attention to the speaker than to himself. This is a training technique, not a therapy technique. Yet it is useful to help you learn how to hear, understand, and accept your patient. Making judgments about your patient creates distant between you and prevents you from hearing what he is trying to say.

Thinking for the Person

Thinking of alternatives and solutions for a patient's problems while he is talking denies him the chance to solve his own problems. This reinforces his feelings of worthlessness and incompetence and sets you up in the advice-giving business. If your patient takes your advice and succeeds, he may discount his accomplishment because "I didn't really do it all by myself." If your suggestions lead to failure, your patient may say, "You gave me bad advice!" In both cases the patient's dependence on others and feelings of ineffectiveness are reinforced. Solving your patient's problems gives the message that you think him incapable of coming to his own solutions. While you are busy planning his solutions, you are missing what he is saying.

Thinking Ahead of the Person

Rushing your patient through his story or trying to get just the facts without the details gives the impression that you are too busy to listen, disinterested, or rude. Listening to the details and context of the situation in full gives you rich opportunities to understand your patient more completely. If your patient speaks tangentially or in fragments, redirect him kindly and gently to the topic. Cutting your patient off can leave him feeling uncared for, unheard, and frustrated. You are not hearing what he is saying if you are thinking of how to interrupt hm.

Listening Distortions

Nichols describes many of the same blocks to effective listening but, in addition, notes that pretending to be attentive, outlining everything that is said, daydreaming, or overreacting to particular words or phrases also interferes with clearly receiving the message that the patient is trying to send [30]. Purtillo suggests that not only are messages blocked by ineffective listening, but they are also distorted in several ways [31].

1. *Mind set.* Your past experiences create a particular set of expectations for what is said in given situations. Your mind is set. That is normal, but you fail to hear your patient's unique differences if you decide in advance that you know what he is going to say. For example, suppose you use the same excuse several times when you get home later than you are expected. "Dad, we ran out of gas." When you really do run out of gas, your dad is not willing to listen. He already knows what you are going to say.

2. *Perceptual defense.* Past experiences also form a familiar context for understanding new ideas. Again that is natural and often helpful, but it is easy to ignore ideas that do not fit your personal situation. Thus you do not hear all of what your patient is trying to tell you. Perceptual defenses lead to rigidity and stereotyping. Snap judgments are easy to make and often lead one astray. In one of *Aesop's Fables,* "The Hare and the Hound," a hound startles a hare from his lair [41]. After a long run the hound gives up the chase. A goatherd seeing him stop mocks him saying, "The little one is the best runner of the two." The hound replies, "You do not see the difference between us. I was only running for a dinner, but he, for his life."

3. *Sensory overload.* The rate of processing information can be influenced by many factors such as external noises and distractions, internal feelings, and physical health. There are times when you cannot concentrate very well. You may be thinking about a new person you just met, remembering what a friend said, or wondering if your headache will go away soon. Your attention is often diverted from your patient to yourself, and you are prevented from hearing what he's saying.

Effective listening occurs only when you are paying attention to your patient instead of yourself. As you talk with your patient, you may find yourself thinking about what you should do or say next. But every second that you are thinking about the right response, you are missing something that your patient is trying to tell you. Should you be concerned with what you say or do? Yes, but not when your patient is talking. Benjamin in *The Helping Interview* eloquently describes this process [5].

When you really listen, almost inevitably a moment's silence will intervene between the interviewee's pausing and your carrying on. Whatever you say or do next will be unpremeditated. It may not be polished or carefully thought through, but it will be genuine. It will come forth spontaneously as the result of your having truly listened. At any rate, you will not have planned your action at the expense of having lost track of the interviewee. You will not sound like the "ideal" interviewer, but you may well sound like yourself. The ideal interviewer does not exist, but you do; and if the interviewee can sense the genuine, unplanned, spontaneous you, he will have an experience rare in our society.

Listening with Your Eyes

Effective listening is facilitated by good observation skills. You need to add what you hear to what you see to understand your patient's meaning. If someone says to you, "You're bad!" you would look at him to see if he were smiling, and you would pay attention to the tone of his voice to see if it held admiration before feeling offended. In the same way, you need to observe your patient's nonverbal expression of his feelings, his tone of voice, and his congruence to determine his meaning.

Nonverbal Expression of Feelings

All of us express our feelings in nonverbal ways. In addition to the body language clues with which you may be familiar, there are other nonverbal indicators about your patient's feelings. Erect posture requires energy to maintain and can indicate that your patient is feeling good. Slumped, slouched posture, however, can indicate a low energy level and feeling down. Good grooming requires investment of energy in oneself. Poor grooming can indicate a lack of energy or inability to invest energy in oneself or both. Pay attention to the nonverbal behaviors associated with particular feelings in your next conversations with your friends; you will be surprised at what you already know.

Tone of Voice

All verbal messages have both the content of what is said and the tone of voice that is used. The tone is crucial in determining what is meant. You probably can recall the exact way your mother's voice sounded when there was no more fooling around; it really was time to go to bed. The same words can hold many meanings depending on how they are spoken. Steve Martin does a comedy routine in which he expresses the entire range of emotions while just repeating "What the hell's going on." Try it out, and notice how the meaning changes when you emphasize different words. Can you express at least 10 different meanings?

Congruence

Is your patient's tone of voice and nonverbal expression congruent with what he is saying? Does he say that everything is "just fine" in a flat tone of voice while sitting slumped in the chair? Incongruence is itself an indicator of a person having trouble [8]. Noticing incongruities is important for two reasons: (1) they help you understand your patient's experience more completely, and (2) handled correctly, they provide excellent opportunities for your patient to grow. Helping, however, must also mean not hurting [8]. Observations are most meaningful when shared as your patient is ready to hear them. See "feedback" (pp. 26–28) in the "responding" section of this chapter for further discussion of this topic.

Improving Your Listening

How can you improve your ability to listen? Reik in his classic work, *Listening with the Third Ear,* suggests that listening can be improved by developing a commitment to listening, avoiding distractions, waiting before responding, and suspending judgments [32]. Smith lists the various levels of listening and proposes that a therapist has difficulty when he fails to match his level of listening to that required in the situation [6].

1. *Analytical.* Listening for specific kinds of information and arranging them into categories.
2. *Directed.* Listening in order to get answers to specific questions.
3. *Attentive.* Listening for general information in order to get the overall picture.

4. *Exploratory.* Listening because of one's own interest in the subject being discussed.
5. *Appreciative.* Listening for esthetic pleasure, such as listening to music.
6. *Courteous.* Listening because one feels obliged to listen.
7. *Passive.* Listening as in overhearing something; not attentive to the matter being discussed.

Most of all, you can improve your listening skills by becoming aware of which blocks and distortions you use the most. Are there particular situations or people that trigger your blocks and distortions? (These require extra attention.) Are you able to concentrate on your patient rather than thinking about what you are going to say next? How are your observation skills? Can you identify nonverbal expressions, tone of voice, and congruence? Are you aware of your different listening levels? Self-assessment of your strengths and problem areas is the first step to improvement.

Your Turn
Recall a conversation you have had recently and look critically at how well you listened. Did you use any of the blocks or distortions? In what way did they affect the conversation? Did you observe nonverbal expression and tone of voice? Did you notice any incongruities? Was your level of listening adequate for the situation?

My listening strengths:

My listening weaknesses:

My plan for change:

Pick one skill that you need to improve, and consciously work on it in conversations with your friends. You will be pleasantly surprised at your results.

Summary
In this section you have been introduced to techniques for active listening and to blocks and distortions that get in the way. By using effective listening skills, you are improving communication with your patient and modeling techniques for him to use. Listening is absolutely necessary for understanding. Active listening demonstrates empathy and gives you the information needed for the next step—responding.

Responding

Charlie Brown: I'm sick of your sly digs! If you don't like me, why don't you come right out and say so!
Lucy: I don't like you.
Charlie Brown: On second thought, I think I prefer the sly digs!

Charles Schultz

By now you are prepared for your patient, you are working with him, you are attending to him nonverbally by watching your eye contact and back channels, you are nurturing him, and you are actively listening to him. Terrific? You have learned your lessons well. There will come a time, however, when you will have to say something. You may wish for a list of just the right things to say, but this is often prompted by the myth that there is only one right response for each situation. Every response is only as effective as how well it is used in that particular context. You not only need to develop a repertoire of response formats, but you also need to develop an appreciation for when to use which one.

Social Chitchat

Social chitchat keeps the conversation superficial, and it diverts attention from your patient to yourself. Social chitchat uses both unrelated and tangential responses [29].

Unrelated Reponses

These responses introduce a subject that is completely different from the one initiated by your patient.

Patient: My mother is very worried that I'm in the hospital.
Therapist: Have you been to see the exhibit at the art center yet?

You have had these conversations. One moment you are talking about cheddar cheese and the next you are talking about vacations in Greece. Associations between the topics are generally not obvious, and if both people do not mind the potpourri of topics unrelated responses are not harmful. If your patient really wants to concentrate on one particular topic, however, unrelated responses can portray you as insensitive and unwilling to talk.

Tangential Responses

These originate from a word or thought contained in your patient's statement, but direct the discussion away from his original purpose.

Patient: My mother is very worried that I'm in the hospital.
Therapist: Mothers are a problem sometimes. Mine called last night and is pressuring me to come home more often.

This response starts out as an attempt to show your patient that you understand what he is talking about, but it changes the focus of attention from his problem to your problem. Used in extremes, tangential responses become insufferable one-upmanship. "You think that's bad? When that happened to me, I thought that I would just die!" You probably can recall the feeling this type of statement evokes.

Unrelated and tangential responses are cocktail party talk. As you mingle, you run through a variety of topics until you find one that you and others can talk about. In that context they are appropriate and useful, but in therapeutic settings they generally are not.

Your Turn

Most definitive statements have at least one exception. In the following space, write about one situation with your patient in which an unrelated or tangential response would be appropriate? (See Selecting Responses, p. 31.)

Paraphrasing

Learning to paraphrase is awkward for most people, yet it is a skill that helps your patient feel accepted, heard, understood, and encouraged. paraphrasing is not repeating his statement to him. Rather, it is trying to capture the essence of his statement and phrasing it in your own words as a way of expressing your sincere desire to understand. Paraphrasing is offering your version of what your patient said. It is useful only in helping to clarify his thoughts and feelings, not in proving that your rendition is the correct one.

Anthony and Carkhuff, from their work with training helpers, suggest that paraphrasing has four levels, which, in developmental order, are (1) responding to the immediate situation, (2) responding to the meaning, (3) responding to the feeling, and (4) responding to the reason for the feeling [8,9]. By upping your response one level at a time, you encourage your patient to explore his feelings in more depth.

Response to the Immediate Situation

Paraphrase the content of your patient's statement to clarify the facts of his situation. Your response might start with "So you're saying . . .?" "You're saying that . . . ?"

Patient: I don't know what to do about my father. He never sems to be satisfied with anything that I do. I feel like such a disappointment to him.
Therapist: So you're saying that you think your father expects too much of you and you're feeling like a disappointment to him?

When your patient has difficulty volunteering the details of the situation, you may use who, what, where, when, and how questions to clarify points. Notice that why is not included as an acceptable question; it is discussed later in this section (see p. 25). Make an effort to intersperse your questions with responses to the immediate situation. This provides more support and prevents your patient from feeling interrogated.

Patient: I don't know what to say next.
Therapist: What did you father say the last time you talked to him?
Patient: It's not so much what he says, but what he doesn't say that gets me. When I told him I was in the hospital, he said, "Well, if you think it's for the best." Then he sighs like he's so disappointed.
Therapist: You're saying that what your father says and how he seems to feel are two different things?

Response to the Meaning

With this response you are not only paraphrasing the content of your patient's response, but you are also trying to identify the meaning that experience holds for him. You attempt to communicate that you are hearing what your patient is saying as well as what he is meaning. This is not an easy task, because the meaning is not always explicit. It is reflected in his nonverbal behavior, his tone of voice, and the content of his statement. No one can or should try to pluck meaning out of thin air; that is mind reading. You need to rely heavily on your understanding of your patient and his statement to determine his meaning. Use your listening and observing skills to determine your patient's meaning, and then treat it as a hypothesis to be verified or refuted. Trying to prove your meaning is the right one to your patient gains you nothing but resentment and passivity.

Your responses might start, "You mean . . .?" or "Do you mean that . . .?"

Patient: I wish it didn't matter so much to me what my father thinks.
Therapist: You mean you'd like to make decisions on your own without worrying about your
    father's opinion.

Response to the Feeling

Paraphrase your patient's statement to identify the specific feelings he has about this situation. "Feelings are the heart of [your patient's] experience of the world. For better or worse, human feelings are perhaps the most fundamental characteristics of human experience." [9, p. 75]. You can attempt to understand your patient's feelings by trying to put yourself in his situation and imagining how you might feel in his spot; however, this is just a start. Some situations represent universal themes and evoke similar feelings in all of us; however, other feelings are idiosyncratic. Use your knowledge of your own feelings only as a place to start to understand your patient, not to tell him how he is feeling. "I know how you feel" is not helpful, because it is not true: You can only know for sure how you feel. You might intend to show that you are trying to understand, but you are implying that there is no need to talk about his feelings further, because you already know how he feels. You are putting up a barrier between you and the patient.

Feelings are of many types and levels of intensity. Very often your patient has difficulty specifying what his feeling is; it may seem vague and undefinable in his mind. By establishing a repertoire of feeling words, you can help your patient clearly identify what he is experiencing. A patient who may appear to be feeling bad may really be feeling hopeless. Table 1-1 lists three levels of intensity for each of seven common emotions [9]. This chart is not inclusive; however, it points out the large range of intensity of feelings. There is a big difference between feeling unsure and feeling trapped. By familiarizing yourself with these different emotion words, you can help your patient express what he is feeling. Your responses might begin with "You're feeling . . . ?" or "Are you feeling . . . ?"

Table 1-1. Categories of feelings

Levels of intensity	Feelings*						
	Happy	Sad	Angry	Confused	Scared	Weak	Strong
Strong	Excited	Hopeless	Furious	Numb	Terrified	Ashamed	Powerful
	Great	Lost	Disgusted	Trapped	Afraid	Vulnerable	Potent
	Overjoyed	Crushed	Enraged	Panicky	Fearful	Exhausted	Aggressive
Mild	Alive	Lonely	Frustrated	Doubtful	Shaky	Embarrassed	Tough
	Proud	Hurt	Irritated	Mixed-up	Worried	Helpless	Confident
	Up	Upset	Sore	Uncomfortable	Anxious	Powerless	Brave
Weak	Calm	Down	Annoyed	Unsure	Nervous	Tired	Healthy
	Glad	Bad	Mad	Surprised	Shy	Shakey	Firm
	Pleased	Dull	Uptight	Foggy	Uneasy	Worn-out	Able

*In order of intensity from bottom to top.
Source: From R. R. Carkhuff, et al., *The Skills of Helping: An Introduction to Counseling Skills*, Amherst, MA: Human Resource Development, 1979. P. 77.

Patient: Just once, I'd like to make a decision without feeling like I had to check it out with my dad.
Therapist: Are you feeling uneasy about making a decision on your own?
Patient: I'm afraid that I'll make the wrong decision without his advice.

Response to the Reason for the Feeling

Paraphrase your patient's statement to help him identify the immediate reason for his feeling. Many feelings have obvious and rational reasons; anyone in the same situation would feel the same way. In other cases, there seems to be no reasonable explanation for one's feelings. Perhaps you have had a day when you felt blue for some reason, but you are not sure why. Anthony and Carkhuff suggest that regardless of how it first appears feelings always turn out to have a sufficient and rational reason [9]. Listen carefully, and try to pinpoint the reason for your patient's feeling from his perspective. His reason does not have to be your reason in order to be sufficient and rational. Pinpointing the reason behind the feeling is important because it prevents your patient from doing something he would like to do, and that is usually the crux of his unhappiness. Your responses might begin "You're feeling . . . [emotion word] because you can't . . . [reason] and you would like to . . . [what it is preventing him from doing]."

Patient: Sometimes I feel so weak.
Therapist: *You're feeling* powerless *because you can't* seem to make decisions on your own, *and you'd like to be* independent?

If you have trouble identifying the reason behind the feeling, drop back to a lower level of paraphrasing until the reason becomes apparent. This pattern of paraphrasing is hierarchical: One step is built on another. So too is the level of trust and mutual respect that grows out of your interaction. During the course of your conversation you may go back and forth between these responses as new topics are introduced and worked through this sequence.

Your Turn

Write a response at each of the four levels of paraphrasing for the following comments. Only the content is provided; you will have to imagine the person's nonverbal behaviors and tone of voice.

1. I hate it when my kids fight with each other. It makes me feel so lousy.

Response to the immediate situation:

Response to the meaning:

Response to the feeling:

Response to the reason for the feeling:

2. I don't really know what I want to do with my life or where I want to go professionally. I thought being an occupational therapist was the thing for me, but now I'm not so sure.

   Response to the immediate situation:

   Response to the meaning:

   Response to the feeling:

   Response to the reason for the feeling:

Questions

As most beginning therapists discover, you'll find that the ability to ask questions in an empathetic and effective manner is a skill you need to develop. Questions can be helpful in obtaining information and clarifying meaning, but they can be overdone. Benjamin challenges the extensive use of the question in therapeutic interactions and suggests that we ask too many meaningless questions that confuse, that cannot possibly be answered, and to which we do not really want to hear the answer [5]. Understanding the different types of questions help us use them more effectively. Questions can be classified by their format, sequence, and effectiveness.

Format

Format refers to the way a question is phrased. In general, all questions can be classified as either open or closed [5].

OPEN QUESTIONS

These questions are very broad in nature and specify only the general topic to be covered. "Tell me something about yourself," or "How are you feeling? are both open questions. Open questions can be further refined into two types: direct or indirect. Open-direct questions are straightforward and restrict the focus of the answer. "How does school seem to you after a week?" or "How do you like to spend your time?" or "Describe yourself as a family member" are all open-direct questions. Open-indirect questions generally have no question mark and inquire without seeming to do so. "Tell me what it's like" or "describe yourself" are open-indirect questions. They show interest, but do not always seem like questions.

Open questions have several advantages. Your patient does most of the talking, and he determines the nature and amount of information he discloses. Open questions are easy to answer and generally pose minimal threat to your patient, because he has control of the information he gives. Open questions also demonstrate your interest in him and can help to establish rapport. Because they are deliberately vague, open questions may elicit information about which you did not think to ask.

Open questions also have several disadvantages. They take skill to use, and because they are vague and unfocused it is easy for your patient to go off on tangents. Open questions also encourage the patient to give you so much information you have difficulty knowing which direction to take.

CLOSED

Closed questions are very restrictive in nature; thus, they limit your patient's answers. "How many brothers and sisters do you have?" or "What time is your next appointment with Dr. Freud?" are both closed questions. Questions that can be answered either yes or no are closed questions, for example, "Are you employed at present?" and "Do you have any children?"

Closed questions have several advantages. You can ask more questions in a short period since the answers are brief, and you have more control of the direction of the conversation. With closed questions, you can get to the facts directly without hoping your patient will volunteer the information.

There are also several disadvantages to closed questions. They tend to polarize opinions, and they do not leave room for gray areas. Because they are so restrictive, you often get too little information, or the answers tend to be superficial and unrevealing about your patient's feelings. Closed questions also do not give him much of a chance to volunteer potentially valuable information. Neither open nor closed questions are the best; however, both have appropriate uses.

Your Turn

Put an O-I before the open-indirect questions, an O-D before the open-direct questions, and a C before the closed questions.

_____ 1. Who brought you to the hospital?
_____ 2. Please tell me what your family is like?
_____ 3. What do you do for a living?
_____ 4. What are your goals?
_____ 5. Do you know what occupational therapy is?
_____ 6. I'd like to hear about what led you to seek treatment at this time.

For the previous six questions rewrite the open questions as closed questions, and the closed questions as both open-direct and open-indirect questions.

1.

2.

3.

4.

5.

6.

7.

8.

Do you think you have it? One more question. Is "What do you want to be when you grow up?" open or closed?

Sequence

In addition to considering the format of questions, you also need to think about their sequence, or the order in which you ask them [5].

PRIMARY

Primary questions introduce a new topic or a new area within a topic. All the questions given as examples so far in this section are primary questions.

SECONDARY

Secondary or follow-up questions are used to elicit more information or develop a single topic more clearly. "Tell me more about . . . " or "What happened then?" or "What did you do after the dog tore the seat out of your pants?" are all secondary questions. Secondary questions are used to help your patient be specific and to explore his feelings about a certain topic area. Asking many questions in a row, however, can leave your patient feeling interrogated, overwhelmed, and defensive. As discussed earlier (p. 17), paraphrasing between questions gives your patient your message of acceptance and willingness to help.

The following example illustrates how primary, secondary, open, and closed questions work together in an interview sequence.

Therapist: Tell me about your educational background (primary, open-direct).
Patient: I graduated from Quest High School and spent two and a half years at college.
Therapist: You're saying you went directly from high school to college?
Patient: Yes, I did.
Therapist: What was your major field of study in college? (secondary, closed).

Patient: I started out in liberal arts and then transferred to engineering.
Therapist: I wonder what college was like for you (secondary, open-indirect).

Your Turn

Following are several topics you might discuss with your patients. For each topic, write a primary and four secondary questions in a logical sequence that would help your patient develop the topic. Include open-direct, open-indirect, and closed questions.

1. Patient's leisure interests

    Primary:

    Secondary:

    Secondary:

    Secondary:

    Secondary:

2. Patient's self-assessment of strengths and weaknesses

    Primary:

    Secondary:

    Secondary:

    Secondary:

    Secondary:

These questions are listed in a row, and asking them in this fashion would bombard and overwhelm your patient. What else do you need to do to increase your rapport and understanding?

Effectiveness

Three types of questions are not effective and should be strictly avoided: double questions, directed questions, and why questions [5].

DOUBLE

Double questions include more than one question at a time. They force a choice between the options stated or confuse the listener.

Therapist: Did you go to occupational therapy yesterday or didn't you?
Patient: Yes.

This exchange was pointless because you still do not know whether your patient attended O.T. Because it conveys a somewhat accusatory message, avoid the "did you or didn't you" format.

Therapist: Would you rather bake a cake or cookies today?
Patient: Neither.

This forced-choice type of double question is often used to limit choices for a patient unable to make decisions, and it is phrased to encourage the person not to take the third option, which is neither. Nonetheless, forced-choice questions are not an effective treatment strategy. It is apparent that you are forcing a choice without acknowledging that you are doing so. Your patient is likely to take the challenge you offer by responding "neither," or by retreating from the challenge and becoming passive, responding, "I don't know." A more effective way to limit choices follows:

Therapist: I think baking is a good activity for you to do today. It will give you practice in doing things step by step. It won't take too long to finish, and you can have it with lunch. You can make either a cake or cookies. Which would you prefer?

This wording presents the two choices along with your reasoning behind them. It limits the options, but gives your patient as much choice as he can handle.

Multiple questions are many questions asked in a row without allowing the listener time to answer.

Therapist: What do you think about the weather today? Do you think your community group will go down to the farmer's market? Is everyone in the group going?
Patient: I don't know.

Overwhelming your patient with so many questions at once is confusing, usually elicits no information, and may damage the rapport you have already established.

DIRECTED

Directed questions suggest (either implicitly or explicitly) the answer you expect to hear. Your patient either agrees or winds up in a no-win position. "Do you dislike the new administrator like most other people I've talked to?" pretty clearly states the answer you expect to hear. Some patients may answer "yes" just to please you, but you still would not know for sure how they felt about the issue. "Have you stopped stealing?" is another no-win question. If answered yes, it is not clear whether your patient did steal at one time and now has quit or whether he has never stolen. If answered no, it is not clear whether he has never stolen or whether he is still stealing. In short, double and directed questions usually give you no usable information and can be detrimental.

WHY?

Why is rarely a helpful question. Although intended to gather information, it frequently implies disapproval and displeasure. "Why are you late?" "Why did you do that?" or "Why did you quit your job?" imply "Don't do that," "I consider this bad," or "You ought to be ashamed." Your patient may feel threatened and withdraw, attack, or rationalize his feelings. Saying "Why are you so upset?" implies that your patient must know the reason behind his feelings. If that were true, your services would not be needed.

Your Turn

Rewrite the following double questions as single questions:

1. Do you want to knit or sew this morning?

2. Where did you go on your vacation? How was the weather? Were the people friendly?

3. Overall, do you feel you have had the usual ups and downs, or do you feel your past has been exceptionally better or worse than that?

Rewrite the following directed questions as neutral.
1. You are coming to O.T., aren't you?

2. This food we have to eat here is pretty bad, isn't it?

3. Are you still drinking?

Rewrite the following why questions.
1. Why are you living at the YWCA?

2. Why was that?

3. Why are you so depressed?

Despite your best intentions, some double, directed, and why questions escape. This exercise is designed to help you identify your typical questioning style. Engage a friend in a conversation about a topic that really interests you and about which you can ask him questions. For instance, you might ask an older person what his life was like at your age, or you might ask a friend about his new computer. When you are finished, assess your question-asking style. Which things do you do well? Is there anything you need to improve?

1. Which of these questions did you use?
   Open-direct:

   Open-indirect:

   Closed:

   Primary:

   Secondary:

2. Did any of these questions sneak in?
   Double:

   Directed:

   Why:

3. Did you notice any patterns?

4. Did you remember to reflect between questions? (Review Reasons for Feelings, pp. 18–19.)

Feedback

Through feedback we can see how others see us. You need to provide feedback to your patient about his behavior, affect, appearance, performance on a task, or incongruities. Feedback is a way of comparing our internal perceptions with other's perceptions of us. You are all familiar with feedback. Grades, comments on papers, and conferences with your teacher or clinical supervisor are all forms of feedback. As you are also aware, feedback can be helpful, even if it's pointing out your mistakes, or it can be so painful that you discount what is said and just feel hurt. How useful a person finds feedback depends largely on how well it is given, not on how accurate it is [18]. Unless your patient can hear the feedback in a nondefensive manner and understand what you mean by it, he will pay no attention. It is possible to give feedback in a helpful, nonthreatening manner, but it takes sensitivity and practice.

Value judgments affect all the responses you give, but they are particularly troublesome when giving feedback. If your patient's behavior, attitude, or appearance does not fit your idea of what is appropriate (based on your values), you may be tempted to tell him "that's inappropriate" and expect him to change. Your observations of your patient do provide valid feedback; however, mandates for change, either expressed or implied, do not. If you offer the patient your perceptions, which are unavoidably based on your values, the patient can more easily accept your feedback, because you are not requesting that he change anything just to please you. You can share what you see happening and how you see that getting in his way, but what he changes, if anything, is up to him. This is most difficult to remember when your patient's behavior is vastly different from what is right for you. One of the key beliefs of the Neuro-Linguistic Programming philosophy may help you keep a sense of perspective on your patient's troublesome behavior. Any behavior, no matter how bizarre, inappropriate, or self-destructive it may seem, is the best possible choice at that time, in that context [2].

The term *giving feedback* has all too frequently become a mask for "Boy, am I going to tell you what I really think about you now!" Giving feedback is not carte blanche to unlease all your pent-up feelings about the person. There are several rules of thumb that will help you give feedback in a nonaggressive, effective manner [18].

1. *Descriptive rather than evaluative.* "You don't like coming to O.T. anymore" is both evaluative and vague. It is not helpful, because your patient has nothing specific to help him understand what you mean. Sharing your response to a specific behavior is much more helpful. "When you look at your watch just as I start to talk to you, I feel as if I'm boring you."
2. *Specific rather than general.* To tell your patient he is a dominating person is not helpful unless you specifically identify what he did to give you that impression. For instance, the statement, "Just now, when you were talking so loudly, I felt put on the spot to defend myself," is more helpful because it identifies the specific behavior and how it makes you feel.
3. *Possible to change.* All feedback is useless unless the person receiving it can do something about what is being identified. The only thing one can do about the comment "I can't stand it because you're so tall!" is to feel unliked.
4. *Possible to accept or decline.* "Don't call me sonny boy!" implies that your patient must change or you will not like him. "I feel put down when you call me sonny boy" points out how his actions are being received. Your patient has the option to change or not to change. It is not a threat, and there is no need to get into a power struggle.
5. *As immediate as possible.* The most effective feedback is given immediately after the behavior, not several days, months, or years later. Do not store up your ammunition. Feedback beginning with "Do you remember last week when you . . . " is not as helpful as it would have been last week.
6. *Solicited rather than imposed.* Sometimes you need to give feedback when it is not requested. At these times, make sure that your need to give feedback is not greater than your patient's need to receive it. This can happen very easily, especially if you are upset with something your patient has done. Keep in mind that your primary motivation is to help your patient and not to ventilate your feelings. Angry feedback is useless.
7. *Small doses.* There is a tendency to save things you wish to discuss and then to talk about them all at once. It is more helpful to present things one at a time, so the patient can think about what you have said.

Positives

Do not forget the positive things the person does. Feedback does not inherently mean things have to change; you do get As on tests sometimes. All feedback is received better if it is preceded by acknowledging the positive, but the positive comments must be sincere, not just a screen for the rest of the feedback to come. "You're pretty smart, for a girl" hides a slap in a seemingly warm comment. "I like you, but I wish you wouldn't . . . " demeans the positive statement by making your acceptance conditional on your patient's change. The same rules apply to positive comments as to other feedback, for example, they should be descriptive, specific, and immediate. Paradoxically, giving positive feedback can sometimes be harmful. Commenting on something that is easy for most people to do, such as making a bed, can be interpreted as a demeaning comment. Even though it may be very difficult for your patient, and you intend to recognize the effort he is putting forth, he may feel that the task should be easy, and your positive feedback reminds him that he is not functioning very well.

Your Turn

As you read through the previous feedback rules you probably thought of a recent interaction in which you were the recipient of the feedback. Did the other person follow the rules? What were your responses? How did the way the feedback was given affect the way you felt?

Recall the last experience you had in which you gave someone feedback. Which of these rules did you use? What was the person's response?

Are there some rules you typically forget to use? (Be honest!)

Rules are fine, but sometimes are hard to apply in real life. The following techniques can help you practice giving effective feedback: (1) owning your messages and (2) understanding the difference between observations and interpretations [38].

Owning Your Messages

I statements rather than *you* statements allow clear and nonaccusatory communication. Saying "I get upset when I hear that," rather than "You upset me when you say that," clearly indicates that you are stating your feelings, thoughts, or wants. You are taking responsibility for your feelings, and you are not blaming your patient for making you feel something. You are acknowledging that your feelings are in your frame of reference and not absolute truths for every one. Owning your feelings not only allows clearer communication, but also models effective communication skills [44].

Your Turn

Circle the following examples in which the speaker owns his message.

1. That makes me furious.
2. We need to meet tomorrow.
3. It seems to me that you have been distant lately.
4. I'm excited about the community group's trip tomorrow.
5. I'm really pleased about your progress.
6. Most people become anxious in these situations.
7. You don't understand me at all.
8. It might be good for the group if we were more open with each other.

9. What's the matter with me?
10. I would appreciate it if you would take this to my office for me.

Change the noncircled statements into *I* statements.

1.

2.

3.

4.

5.

6.

7.

Observation Versus Interpretation

As discussed in the listening section (p. 12), an observation is a description of what your senses perceive—what you can see, taste, touch, smell, and hear. Good observations are made with suspended judgments. For example, "I noticed when you made the drawing of your family you left yourself out" is an observation. Interpretations suggest, state, or presume the meaning your observation holds for the patient. For example, "I notice you aren't in your drawing. You're feeling like you aren't part of your family. You must be really angry with them" is an interpretation. Ultimately, your interpretation may turn out to be true, or it may not be. If it is accurate, you have denied your patient the opportunity to make that discovery for himself. In a way, it is like having someone tell you what happens at a movie just before the end.

When your interpretation is inaccurate, several things can happen. If it is presented as a question, your patient can at least accept or decline it (although that may take a lot of strength). Often, however, interpretations are presented as facts. Your patient may become passive and think, "Well, she's the therapist, she's probably right." On the other hand, your patient might feel offended and defend himself as well as he can, by withdrawing, challenging, or quitting treatment.

Interpretations often carry a judgmental tone. They imply that the patient is wrong, bad, or somehow inadequate and must change, rather than objectively identifying the behavior and then allowing him to make an informed, individual choice. One more example: "Molly, I notice that you've said several times you have a hard time making decisions, and they seem to be connected to when you try new projects. What do you make of that?" is an observation. "Your difficulty in making decisions when you try new things is due to your excessively perfectionist standards and fear of failure" is an interpretation.

Your Turn

Carefully examine each of the following statements. Is it an observation, interpretation, or both? Identify each statement's strong and weak points. Incorporate everything you have learned about asking questions and giving feedback.

1. John, I've noticed that sometimes you hit other people when you lose a game. What is that all about?

2. Why are you angry with me?

3. Sally, your foot is just tapping away. Are you nervous? You're making me nervous.

4. That black paint looks awfully depressing. Are you feeling depressed?

5. Your constant preoccupation with food, calories, and the scale is preventing you from living your life in a fulfilling manner.

6. You're making me frustrated by having me constantly beg you to come to O.T.

7. Jo, that's inappropriate. Please stop.

Selecting Responses

You have been introduced to several responding behaviors in this chapter: paraphrasing, questioning, and providing feedback. With experience, you will be able to recognize situations that call for each type of response and use that response without consciously thinking about it. For a while, however, this process will take practice.

The specific problems your patient experiences influence your selection of responding action. Some responses are more appropriate for some situations than for others. A few examples of common errors are provided for illustration.

Paraphrasing can be more frustrating than helpful when used with a patient with serious cognitive impairments. You both go in circles repeating the same sentence and accomplishing nothing.

Patient: I don't feel like coming to O.T. this morning.
Therapist: So you're saying that you are not coming?

Patient: I don't think that I'll come today.
Therapist: You mean that you're not coming to O.T. today because you don't feel like it?

The only thing that occurs in this interaction is that both of you feel frustrated and unheard. Patients who have previously been in therapy may perceive such an interchange as verbal sparring. It is likely that the patient comprehends what you are saying, but has negative associations with paraphrasing. Spend extra time building rapport with this patient. He needs assurance that you are sincerely trying to understand him.

Responding to the reason for the feeling should not be introduced too quickly with patients experiencing difficulty establishing trust, as it will be interpreted as prying rather than an attempt to understand. For instance:

Therapist: How are things going, Jane?
Patient: Oh, OK I guess.
Therapist: You're looking sad. Any particular reason?
Patient: Every time Dr. Freud talks to me, I feel like this.
Therapist: You mean that when you're through with your therapy appointment, you leave feeling sad?
Patient: I feel alone.
Therapist: Are you feeling vulnerable?
Patient: Yes.
Therapist: You're feeling vulnerable because you've shared private and important things with Dr. Freud and you're not sure what is going to happen next?

This interaction follows the paraphrasing sequence, but leaps to the reason behind the feeling much too quickly. Even if you are sure you know what the reason is, the patient needs to be ready to hear and accept it. This interaction pushed her before she was ready, and it will affect her ability to trust you again. Spend time responding to the meaning and the feelings before you start responding to the reason for the feeling. Monitor your patient's reactions carefully and be prepared to drop back to the other levels of responding. It is not realistic to expect each interaction you have with a patient to reach the reason-behind-the-feeling level. Not all interactions must end at this level to be considered effective and productive.

A patient experiencing circumstantiality, distractability, illogical thinking, loose associations, or pressure of speech can often be refocused on the task by using closed questions and tangential responses. However, be sure to preface this refocusing with a statement explaining what you are doing. Otherwise, the rapport you have developed so far will be damaged.

Patient: . . . and he couldn't believe that this was really happening.
Therapist: We seem to have gotten on to another topic, and I wanted to hear more about your job. Do you work alone?
Patient: . . . my dad was really happy.
Therapist: You mentioned your dad, and let's talk about your relationship with him . . .

These responses acknowledge that you heard your patient, but still help you maintain some direction in the interview. Using open questions would only encourage further wandering from the topic and facilitate expression of your patient's symptoms. That would be painful for him and unproductive for both of you.

Your Turn
What other types of patient problems could have an influence on the type of responding you would select? State the preferred response for each one.

Problems   *Preferred responses*

_____   _____

_____   _____

_____   _____

_____   _____

_____   _____

_____   _____

Summary

In this section you have been introduced to the use of paraphrasing, questions, and feedback as responding skills. The cookbook "right response" does not exist, but the techniques presented can help you increase your skills and confidence in responding to your patient. The final step is to try these new skills.

Comedian: Say, do you know how I get to Carnegie Hall?
Straight man: Practice! Practice! Practice!
Old vaudeville routine

If the meaning of any communication is the response it elicits, regardless of your intention [2], then it is not enough just to read about developing better communication skills. With enough practice, the communication skills you have just read about will become integrated. You will not have to think about what you need to do next when you are working with a patient. These skills will become part of your style; indeed, part of you.

One of the most common situations employing all of these skills is the interview. Interviews are defined as a conversation between two people that is serious and purposeful [45]. They are used extensively by occupational therapists working in psychiatry as a method of assessment. In fact, Hemphill found that 75 percent of the psychiatric occupational therapists she surveyed used the interview as their only method of assessment [20]. Being able to interview well is a skill you will need.

Interviews can be very structured (with a standardized list of questions allowing no deviation), unstructured (with no predetermined questions or direction), or somewhere in between (semistructured) [21]. In most assessment interviews, many topics are addressed superficially in a short time; thus responding actions that focus and limit your patient's responses are useful.

Interviews progress through three phases: opening, body, and closing [5].

1. *Opening.* The first few minutes of the interview are a good opportunity for building rapport. Let your patient know what to expect by informing him of the purpose of the interview and how long you have to talk. Start with getting-to-know-you questions about such demographic data as age and educational background. Your preparing and attending skills are important at this phase to help fully engage your patient in the interview.

2. *Body.* The major work of the interview is done in this phase. Use your attending, listening, and responding skills to help your patient answer questions and identify the issues you will work on together. Interviews can become choppy and fragmented if many topics are covered. Remember to use secondary questions for each primary question posed, and make the transitions from one topic to another as unobtrusive as possible.

3. *Closure.* Allow a little time before the end to summarize the major themes discussed, wrap up the discussion, and offer your patient the opportunity to ask you questions. This is not the time to introduce new material; everything summarized should have been addressed in the preceding discussion. Should the patient bring up a new topic at this point, acknowledge it, and make arrangements to discuss it later. If it is a topic that needs immediate attention and your schedule does not permit the extra time, arrange for follow-up from another staff member.

Your last assignment for this chapter is to conduct a tape-recorded interview. If you have the equipment readily available, a video recording is even better; however, an audio recording is less threatening and will suffice. Recording your interview gives you the chance to be a Monday-morning quarterback; you will be able to assess the skills you perform well and those you need to work on further. This interview will not only provide you with the opportunity to collect and interpret data in the areas of occupational role status and balance, but it will also provide you with the chance to practice your communication skills. Interview an acquaintance rather than a patient for this assignment. You need the opportunity to try your new skills in this first interview without any special patient problem to handle. Your subject should answer questions as he normally would and not try to pretend to be a patient. This will give you the most accurate and realistic information.

If this assignment is for a class, ask your subject to sign the release form (Fig. 1-1), and turn it in with the tape to your instructor. In any case, tell your subject what is going to happen to the tape and who, if anyone, will listen to it. Tips for getting a good-quality audio recording are listed in Table 1-2.

Instrument

The interview format provided for you to use is adapted from the Occupational Role History Interview (ORHI), developed by Florey and Michelman [16]. It is based on the model of human occupation frame of reference, and it yields information about role performance that is useful for all frames of reference. Before you begin, familiarize yourself with the protocol for using this interview and interpreting the data.

Three occupational roles are addressed by the ORHI: worker, homemaker, and student. Role status refers to how well the subject has met the responsibilities of his occupational roles over time. That is, how well has he performed in role(s) in the past and how well is he performing now. Role balance refers to the balance of your subject's leisure activities and the activities required for his occupational role. In other words, does your subject have a balance between his leisure activities and his

Fig. 1-1. Release form for audio taping of voice.

I agree to participate in an interview with _____
(student's name)

that is tape recorded for educational use in _____
(name of class)

at _____ on _____
(name of school)   (date)

_____   _____
(subject's signature)   (printed name)

_____
(street address)

_____   _____   _____
(city)   (state)   (zip)

_____
(signature of student)

_____
(date)

Student: Please turn this form in with your tape recording.

Table 1-2. Tips for a good quality recording

1. Choose a quiet, distraction-free environment. You and the subject will be able to relax more if you have privacy.
2. Use a 90-minute tape (45 min on each side) so you will not have to turn it over.
3. Do not start to record until the tape runs past the blank leader tape. Let the tape run for several seconds to make sure.
4. Push the *play* and *record* buttons simultaneously to record. If you use an external microphone, make sure the *off/on* switch is set to *on*.
5. Set the sound level. Keep the microphone about four to six inches from your subject's mouth. Position the microphone on a table in front of your subject and leave it alone. Do not hold it in your hand or stick it in front of your subject's face, reporter style.
6. Relax, smile, and try to forget that you are taping.

work, homemaking, or school activities? (Criteria for determining role status and role balance are described under "Interpretation," p. 36.)

Administration

The ORHI (see Fig. 1-2) is designed for use with young-adult to middle-aged subjects. It is a semistructured interview, so you may add or delete questions as you find necessary. This interview is an opportunity to practice all your communication skills, from attending to responding. Before you begin, think about how each of these skills will apply in this interview situation. For example, asking your subject to participate in this assignment is similar to getting your patient to participate in O.T. As with a patient, the way you state your request will largely determine your success or failure in getting the subject involved.

Fine a quiet, private place for your interview, and gather all the supplies you will need in advance (taping materials, coffee, release form). Review the questions, and note that a different sequence of questions is used for the student role than for the homemaker and worker roles. Familiarize yourself with the topics, and anticipate additional secondary questions that might be useful. You do not need to take notes; you have the tape recorder. Your attending and listening skills become sharper when you do not rely on notes. Finally, review the hints for making a good tape recording (Table 1-2) and you are ready to start!

Demographic data
Name:
Age:
Sex:
Educational level:
Occupational role(s):

For worker and homemaker, ask the following questions:
1. What is your current occupation?
2. How did you choose this occupation?
3. What kind of tasks does it include?
4. How did you learn the daily routine?
5. What do you like about what you are doing?
6. What do you dislike about what you are doing?
7. What are you good at?
8. What are your problem areas?
9. How many other jobs or occupations have you had?
   a. What were they?
   b. How did you go about getting them?
   c. What job did you hold the longest?
   d. What was your favorite job?
10. Is there anyone you admire or want to be like now and in the past?
11. What kind of work do your parents do?
12. Did your parents have any influence on your choice of occupation?
13. When do you do your chores?
14. How do you spend your leisure time?
15. What do you do for fun?
16. Do you have any hobbies?
17. What interests would you like to explore?
18. Do you have any close friends? How often do you see them?
19. What do you do together?
20. What was the best period in your life? What was happening then?
21. What was the worst period in your life? What was happening then?
22. What would you like to be doing a year from now?
23. How will you go about doing that?

Fig. 1-2. Suggested questions for use in the Occupational Role History Interview. (Modified from L. L. Florey and S. M. Michelman, Occupational role history: A screening tool for psychiatric occupational therapy. Am. J. Occup. Ther. 36:301, 1982.)

Fig. 1-2 (continued)

24. How would you assess your ability to meet your responsibilities as a _____? (patient's occupation)
25. Are you satisfied with your performance?
26. Do you have a balance of leisure and work activities at the present time?
27. Is that satisfactory?

For the student, ask the following questions:
1. What school(s) did you go to?
2. How did you do in school?
3. What did you like about school?
4. What did you not like about school?
5. What were you good at in school?
6. What were your problem areas?
7. What did you major in? How did you decide on that major?
8. Whom did you admire during that period?
9. Did you have any favorite teachers?
10. What kinds of things did you do for fun?
11. Where did you live during that time?

If the student has had any part-time or summer employment, ask the following questions.
If the student has no work experience, skip to question 24.
12. What is your current occupation?
13. How did you choose this occupation?
14. What kind of tasks does it include?
15. How did you learn the daily routine?
16. What do you like about what you are doing?
17. What do you dislike about what you are doing?
18. What are you good at?
19. What are your problem areas?
20. How many other jobs or occupations have you had?
    a. What were they?
    b. How did you go about getting them?
    c. What job did you hold the longest?
    d. What was your favorite job and why?
21. Is there anyone you admire or want to be like, now and in the past?
22. What kind of work do your parents do?
23. Did your parents have any influence on your choice of occupation?
24. When do you do your chores?
25. How do you spend your leisure time?
26. What do you do for fun?
27. Do you have any hobbies?
28. What interests would you like to explore?
29. Do you have any close friends? How often do you see them?
30. What do you do together?
31. What was the best period in your life? What was happening then?
32. What was the worst period in your life? What was happening then?
33. What would you like to be doing a year from now?
34. How will you go about doing that?
35. How would you assess your ability to meet your responsibilities as a _____? (patient's occupation)
36. Are you satisfied with this performance?
37. Do you have a balance of leisure and work activities at the present time?
38. Is that satisfactory?

Interpretation

At the conclusion of the interview, reflect on the information you received and assess your subject's functioning in two areas: role status and role balance.

Role Status

Role status is the ability to meet the responsibilities of the worker, homemaker, or student role, and can be rated as functional, temporarily impaired, or dysfunctional.

1. *Functional.* Describes a subject who has had a pattern of successful performance of role responsibilities in the past and continues to perform successfully. The quality of his performance can range from adequate to excellent, but his pattern is consistent in meeting his role responsibilities.
2. *Temporarily impaired.* Describes a subject who has performed his role responsibilities successfully in the past, but is currently having difficulty meeting these responsibilities.
3. *Dysfunctional.* Describes a subject whose performance of role responsibilities has been inadequate or sporadic in the past. He is continuing to have difficulty performing these responsibilities. Because you are unable to observe your subject's actual performance of his role responsibilities, you have to base your rating on his report. Compare his self-assessment with the historical information, and note if there is any inconsistency.

Role Balance

Role balance is your subject's pattern, over time, of participation in leisure activities that he identifies as different from his work activities. This determination is based on your subject's definitions of work and leisure. For instance, a mechanic might fix automobiles all day and find tinkering with his car at night to be leisure. Or a chef might whip up gourmet meals for fun on the weekend. You may not think that sounds like leisure, but your assessment should reflect your subject's activity values, not yours. You will learn more about interference of your own values in determining a patient's problem areas in the next chapter. Your subject's pattern can be rated as ongoing, sporadic, or absent.

1. *Ongoing.* Describes a subject with a fairly consistent pattern of distinctly different leisure and work activities. The amount of participation in leisure activities may vary over time, but the subject has interests to pursue and is currently involved in leisure activities.
2. *Sporadic.* Describes a subject with occasional participation in leisure activities or occasional differentiation between work and leisure activities. He is currently not involved in any leisure activity. He may have leisure interests, but is not pursuing them at present.
3. *Absent.* Describes a subject with a history of minimal participation in leisure activities or no distinction between work and leisure activities. Subject is currently not involved in any leisure activity and can state no leisure interest.

Finally, rate your subject's level of satisfaction with his ability to meet his role responsibilities and his balance of work and leisure activities. Rate as either satisfied or dissatisfied.

Record your interpretation and your ratings on the form provided. Indicate the basis for your rating by quoting from the interview.

History of role:

Role status (check the one that applies):
_____ functional
_____ temporarily impaired
_____ dysfunctional
Basis for decision:

Role balance (check the one that applies):

_____ ongoing

_____ sporadic

_____ absent

Basis for decision:

Subject's satisfaction with role status: _____ satisfied   _____ dissatisfied

Subject's satisfaction with role balance: _____ satisfied   _____ dissatisfied

Basis for decision:

Self-Evaluation

After you complete the interview and fill out the rating scale, listen to the tape and evaluate yourself on the following checklist. Use this opportunity to pat yourself on the back for the things you did well as well as a chance to identify areas you need to work on further. After your fieldwork, you probably will not have close professional supervision from another occupational therapist. You are ultimately responsible for your own professional growth and development; this can be a good opportunity to start that process.

Occupational Role History Interview Self-Evaluation

Attending skills	_Good_	_Needs work_
1. Preparation of the subject: your introduction of the purpose of the interview	_____	_____
2. Preparation of the setting: physical surroundings private and conducive	_____	_____
3. Attending actions: your positioning, eye contact, and use of back channels	_____	_____
4. Nurturing: use of any nurturing actions	_____	_____
5. Avoidance of listening blocks or distortions	_____	_____
6. Observation skills: tone of voice, nonverbal expression, and congruence	_____	_____
7. Match of listening level to the level required	_____	_____
8. Appropriate use of social chitchat	_____	_____
9. Paraphrasing:		
Appropriate levels	_____	_____
Correct sequence	_____	_____
10. Questions:		
Use of open and closed questions	_____	_____
Use of secondary questions	_____	_____
Avoidance of double, directed, or why questions	_____	_____
11. Use of feedback	_____	_____
12. Progression of the interview: moving from opening, to body, to closing	_____	_____

References

1. Allen, C. K. *Occupational Therapy for Psychiatric Diseases: Measurement and Management of Cognitive Disabilities.* Boston: Little, Brown, 1985.
2. Bandler, R., and Grinder, S. *Frogs Into Princes: Neuro Linguistic Programming.* Moab, UT: Real People, 1979. P. 3.
3. Barris, R. Environmental interactions: An extension of the model of human occupation. *Am. J. Occup. Ther.* 36:637, 1982.
4. Barris, R., Kielhofner, G., and Watts, J. H. *Psychosocial Occupational Therapy: Practice in A Pluralistic Arena.* Laurel, MD: Ramsco, 1983.
5. Benjamin, A. *The Helping Interview* (3rd ed.). Boston: Houghton Mifflin, 1981. P. 109.
6. Brill, N. I. *Working With People: The Helping Process* (2nd ed.). New York: Lippincott and Harper & Row, 1978.
7. Carkhuff, R. R. New directions in training for the helping professions: Toward a technology for human and community resource development. *The Counseling Psychologist* 3:12, 1972.
8. Carkhuff, R. R. *The Art of Helping IV.* Amherst, MA: Human Resource Development, 1980.
9. Carkhuff, R. R., and Anthony, W. A. *The Skills of Helping: An Introduction to Counseling Skill.* Amherst, MA: Human Resource Development, 1979.
10. Clark, P. N. Human development through occupation: Theoretical frameworks in contemporary occupational therapy practice, Part 1. *Am. J. Occup. Ther.* 33:305, 1979.
11. Corry, S., Sebastian, V., and Mosey, A. C. Acute short-term treatment in psychiatry. *Am. J. Occup. Ther.* 28:401, 1971.
12. Dinkmeyer, D., and Losoncy, L. E. *The Encouragement Book: Becoming A Positive Person.* Englewood Cliffs, NJ: Prentice-Hall, 1980.
13. Dunning, H. Environmental occupational therapy. *Am. J. Occup. Ther.* 32:305, 1978.
14. Eagan, G. *The Skilled Helper: A Model for Systematic Helping and Interpersonal Relating.* Monterey, CA: Brooks/Cole, 1975.
15. Fidler, G. S., and Fidler, J. W. Doing and becoming: Purposeful action and self-actualization. *Am. J. Occup. Ther.* 32:305, 1978.
16. Florey, L. L., and Michelman, S. M. Occupational role history: A screening tool for psychiatric occupational therapy. *Am. J. Occup. Ther.* 36:301, 1982.
17. Frazier, S. H., et al. *A Psychiatric Glossary.* New York: Basic Books, 1975.
18. Hanson, P. G. Giving Feedback: An Interpersonal Skill. In J. W. Pfeiffer and J. E. Jones (eds.), *Annual Handbook for Group Facilitators.* La Jolla, CA: University Associates, 1975.
19. Harper, R. G., Wiens, A. D., and Matarayzo, J. D. *Nonverbal Communication: The State of the Art.* New York: Wiley, 1978.
20. Hemphill, B. J. Mental health evaluations used in occupational therapy. *Am. J. Occup. Ther.* 34:721, 1980.
21. Hemphill, B. J. The Evaluation Process. In B. J. Hemphill (ed.), *The Evaluative Process in Psychiatric Occupational Therapy.* Thorofare, NJ: Slack, 1982.
22. Ivey, A., and Authier, S. *Microcounseling.* Springfield, IL: Thomas, 1978.
23. Kannegeiter, R. B. Environmental interactions in psychiatric occupational therapy—Some influences. *Am. J. Occup. Ther.* 34:715, 1980.
24. King, L. J. A sensory-integrative approach to schizophrenia. *Am. J. Occup. Ther.* 28:529, 1974.
25. LaFrance, M., and Mayo, C. *Moving Bodies: Nonverbal Communication in Social Relationships.* Monterey, CA: Brooks/Cole, 1978.
26. Madigan, J. M. Characteristics of students in occupational therapy educational programs. *Am. J. Occup. Ther.* 39:41, 1985.
27. Mosey, A. C. Meeting Health Needs. *Am. J. Occup. Ther.* 27:14, 1973.
28. Mosey, A. C. *Occupational Therapy: Configuration of a Profession.* New York: Raven, 1981.
29. National Institute on Drug Abuse. *The Social Seminar, Drugs, Education and Society: A Resource Manual for the Group Facilitator.* U.S. Dept. of Health, Education, and Welfare, 1975.
30. Nichols, R. G. Listening is good business. *Management Personnel Quarterly* 1:2, 1962.
31. Purtilo, R. *Health Professional/Patient Interaction* (2nd ed.). Philadelphia: Saunders, 1978.
32. Reik, T. *Listening with the Third Ear.* New York: Pyramid, 1972.
33. Reiser, D. E., and Schroder, A. K. *Patient Interviewing: The Human Dimension.* Baltimore: Williams & Williams, 1980. P. 96.
34. Rogers, C. *On Becoming a Person.* Boston: Houghton Mifflin, 1961.

35. Schroeder, C. V., et al. *SBC Adult Psychiatric Sensory Integration Evaluation Manual.* La Jolla, CA: SBC Research Associates, 1978.

36. Smith, E. Improving listening effectiveness. *Tex. Med.* 71:98, 1975.

37. Steward, J. (ed.). *Bridges Not Walls: A Book About Interpersonal Communication.* Menlo Park, CA: Addison Wesley, 1973.

38. Steward, C. J., and Cash, W. G. *Interviewing: Principles and Practices.* Dubuque, IA: William G. Brown, 1974.

39. Sue, S., McKinney, H., and Allen, D. B. Predictors of the duration of therapy for clients in the community mental health center system. *Comm. Men. Health J.* 12:374, 1976.

40. Tiffany, E. G. Psychiatry and Mental Health. In H. L. Hopkins, and H. D. Smith (eds.), *Willard and Spackman's Occupational Therapy* (5th ed.). Philadelphia: Lippincott, 1978.

41. Townsend, G. T. (trans.). *Aesop's Fables.* Garden City, NY: Doubleday, 1968.

42. Truax, C. B., and Carkhuff, R. R. *Toward Effective Counseling and Psychotherapy: Training and Practice.* Chicago: Aldine, 1967.

43. Truax, C. B., and Mitchell, K. M. Research on Certain Therapist Interpersonal Skills in Relation to Process and Outcome. In A. E. Bergin and S. L. Garfield (eds.), *Handbook of Psychotherapy and Behavior Change: An Empirical Analysis.* New York: Wiley, 1971.

44. Wismer, J. N. Communication Effectiveness: Active Listening and Sending Feeling Messages. In J. W. Pfeiffer, and J. E. Jones, (eds.), *Annual Handbook for Group Facilitators.* La Jolla, CA: University Associates, 1978.

45. Zaro, J. S., et al. *A Guide for Beginning Psychotherapists.* New York: Cambridge University Press, 1982.

I can't say . . . that I learned what I had wanted to know because I hadn't known what I wanted to know.

William Least Heat Moon
Blue Highways

Mr. Casey was Jo's first patient. He was a new referral to O.T., so Jo was responsible for executing the entire treatment process. Feeling nervous yet excited, Jo tried to decide what she should do first. *Should I read his chart, or would that bias my judgments?* When she looked at his chart, Jo felt overwhelmed. Mr. Casey had been treated several times before, and his chart was as thick as Willard and Spackman's! *How much of this information is really relevant to what I'm going to do in O.T.?* she thought. Jo knew that she needed to evaluate Mr. Casey before she planned his treatment, but which evaluation should she use? *Should I interview him first? Maybe I should observe his performance in O.T. clinic groups for today. The O.T. department just got a new self-care evaluation; maybe I should use that with Mr. Casey? Perhaps a sensory integration evaluation would be the best. Maybe I can do all of them! Where do I start?*

Jo raised many good questions about the assessment process. Where do you start? The first step is to remind yourself of the entire treatment process [3,79,89,104].

1. *Referral.* Patients are referred to O.T. on a case-by-case basis or on a blanket referral that includes everyone in the treatment program.
2. *Screening.* Preliminary assessment is made of the patient's major problems and his need for O.T. Preliminary problems amenable to O.T. intervention are identified.
3. *Evaluation.* Evaluations of specific problem areas are conducted as indicated. Evaluation data are interpreted. Patient's problems and strengths are described.
4. *Treatment planning.* Goals, objectives, and methods of O.T. intervention are identified.
5. *Treatment implementation.* Intervention is implemented, patient status is re-evaluated, plan is revised as needed, and outcome of treatment is assessed.
6. *Termination of treatment.* Occupational therapy is discontinued when intervention is completed.

Your Turn
Start with a review of the terminology of assessment. Define the following terms in the spaces provided. (Refer to Maurer et al. [74] if you get stuck.)

Assessment:

Evaluation:

Screening:

Instrument:

Objective:

Subjective:

Standardized:

Norms:

Valid:

Reliable:

The Role of Theory

Each time I see the Upside-Down Man
Standing in the water,
I look at him and start to laugh,
Although I shouldn't oughtter.
For maybe in another world
Another time
Another town,
Maybe HE is right side up
And I am upside down.

                                    Shel Silverstein
                                    "Reflection"*

Evaluation of psychiatric disorders is particularly challenging. These disorders create both functional and qualitative problems in living; every aspect of your patient's life conceivably could be evaluated and treated. You do not have time, nor will you be reimbursed, for such major life revisions. One could debate the need for them as well. Somehow the scope of the services you provide must be defined and limited. Lack of distinct parameters to the areas of patient functioning that O.T. treats (our defined domain of concern) creates confusion, both inside and outside the profession. Trying to treat all of your patient's problems fragments your efforts. Work may be started, but not finished leaving both of you wondering what, if anything, was accomplished. The domain of concern thus provides boundaries limiting the areas that occupational therapists are concerned with assessing and treating [79].

At present, no universal agreement exists within the O.T. profession about what our domain of concern should contain [70,80]. Some therapists endorse the generalist approach typified by the American Occupational Therapy Association's (AOTA) Uniform Evaluation Checklist [3], whereas others believe we need more precision, clarity, and limits to our domain of concern [2]. Each frame of reference provides general guidelines for selection of areas to be included in its domain of concern. Nevertheless, we lack specific definition and evidence of the areas that are most successfully treated by O.T. Until we have outcome studies that indicate our effectiveness in treating particular areas of functioning, our selection of areas to include in our domain of concern is based on our philosophy, theoretic assumptions, and clinical judgment. Areas appearing frequently in the literature as part of our domain of concern follow [3,79,89]:

1. Living situation and responsibilities
2. Self-care and personal hygiene
3. Homemaking
4. Work
5. Play and leisure
6. Self-esteem and self-concept
7. Situational coping
8. Self-expression and self-control
9. Cognitive functioning
10. Neuromuscular functioning
11. Sensory integration
12. Interpersonal relationships
13. Environmental constraints and resources

Assessment of each of these areas would generate more information than you would be able to make sense of or do anything about. The boundaries of our domain of concern are, at present, provided by theory. The theoretic frame of reference organizes what is known in a field and describes the relationships between its facts and concepts [69]. It narrows the areas in our domain of concern, defines relationships among these areas, and provides structure for assessment and treatment planning. Mosey describes a frame of reference as consisting of: "(1) a statement of the theoretical base; (2) delineation of function-dysfunction continuums; (3) a listing of behaviors indicative of function and dysfunction; and (4) postulates regarding intervention" [79, p. 133]. Thus, a frame of reference provides systematic guidelines for your interactions with patients. In practice, two occupational therapists treating the same patient but using different frames of reference would identify different areas of the patient's functioning to assess (domain of concern), use different evaluation instruments, use different criteria for interpreting the results of these instruments, and define different problems and strengths relevant to O.T. treatment.

Historically, occupational therapists have applied psychologic theories to their practice; thus, concepts of analytic, behavioral, developmental, and humanistic theories were used as both a rationale and theoretic base for O.T. treatment [23,26, 35,68,77,78,79,99,101]. However well these psychologic theories were understood and applied, they did not completely translate into practical working concepts for O.T. A gap existed between knowledge of the theory and an understanding of how to use it with the patient. Consequently, for many therapists, theory has become disconnected from the work they do every day [58]. Other therapists have found their own ways of integrating theory and practice, resulting in differences and inconsistencies in the type and quality of O.T. services being delivered and creating concern that this fragmentation is getting us off the track, or derailing O.T. [100].

Dissatisfaction with these inconsistencies in treatment, emerging neuroscience literature challenging our "traditional" views, and the rapidly changing arena in which occupational therapists deliver health care services have inspired a growing movement to define and articulate O.T. frames of reference that are distinct from psychologic theories. Several O.T. frames of reference have emerged from this effort. They are compatible with various psychologic theories and borrow elements of them for their own theoretic bases. Yet each represents O.T.'s unique background of biologic sciences, psychology, sociology, arts, medicine, and activities. Each addresses the whole person functioning in his environment, and each provides guidelines for assessment and intervention. Four frames of reference are discussed in this book: (1) functional performance, (2) sensory integration, (3) the model of human occupation, and (4) cognitive disabilities. They are in different stages of development, and much research needs to be completed to expand, test, and validate each one. Yet they represent hope that our unique theoretic base can be refined, articulated, and applied to the treatment of psychiatric disorders.

These frames of reference represent divergent views. However, contrasting views of the nature and treatment of psychiatric disorders are long-standing phenomena. Divergent positions are not unique to O.T., but are shared with other professions. For example, psychology alternates between cycles of fierce competition for acceptance of a new or "superior" theory and attempts to integrate competing theories into a single conceptual scheme [55,93]. Currently, many psychologists are attempting to put aside their rival conceptual positions to find their common ground. This move toward integration was spawned by the recognition of several factors. First, using just one theoretic approach was limiting. Principles of cognitive psychology had become so widely accepted and used by all theoretic approaches that most were no longer pure. Second, theories considered to be in competition were found to have many similarities. Surprisingly, treatment techniques across all theories were, in actual practice, more similar than their theoretic constructs would suggest. Finally, research data indicate that the outcomes produced by different techniques are not obviously different [55].

Occupational therapy has experienced similar cycles of competition for the "superior O.T. theory" and attempts to propose a unifying theory for all of O.T. [27,

32,51,53,56,63,68,90]. As with the field of psychology, commonalities have been identified between seemingly disparate frames of reference [71,72]. Yet despite the apparent differences, common clinical intervention strategies can be identified across all frames of reference. These include the teaching-learning process, purposeful activities, activity groups, activity analysis and synthesis, and conscious use of self. These commonalities, or "legitimate tools of O.T." [79], are explained in Chap. 3.

The emergence of new frames of reference and refinement of familiar ones engenders a tendency to declare exclusive allegiance to one [80]. As our knowledge base develops and the constructs of these frames of reference are validated through research, we may ultimately discard some and wholeheartedly embrace others. Until then, however, familiarity with each frame of reference and rigorous application of their constructs to clinical practice is essential. Eclecticism does not have to mean using an intuitive, nonconceptual approach. There is always the danger that eclecticism can be used to justify a superficial, haphazard approach to patient assessment and treatment. It is also true that lack of commitment to any one frame of reference can mask ignorance of the theoretic basis guiding clinical judgments. Nevertheless, eclecticism can also identify an attitude of willingness to acknowledge, understand, and use the concepts of all frames of reference, regardless of whether one leans toward a preferred one [40]. "At a time of imperfect knowledge, when each of the . . .theoretical foundations . . . offers some answers but none holds them all, it would seem professionally irresponsible for clinicians to do otherwise" [108, p. 31].

The four frames of reference discussed in this book are summarized in the following sections with a focus on the assessment process. They are mentioned for purposes of comparison only; additional study of the constructs of each is required. Consult the references listed at the end of the chapter for more information.

1. *Functional performance.* The purpose of assessment is to identify problems in work, play, or self-maintenance [27,37,79]. It is postulated that these roles are affected by the patient's biologic endowment, maturation, environment, and personal expectations. Dysfunctional behavior therefore must be examined in the context of the patient's age, culture, expectations, and environmental barriers. The presence of dysfunction in work, play, self-maintenance, or in the balance of these roles warrants further assessment of the postulated components underlying performance: sensory integration, motor, psychologic, cognitive, and social functioning [27,33,69]. Standardized instruments, interviews, and clinical observations are used for both screening and evaluation [27,33].

2. *Sensory integration.* The purpose of assessment is to identify the presence of any sensory integrative dysfunction. It is postulated that adequate sensory processing and neural organization is a prerequisite for the patient's effective functioning in daily living skills [49,71]. Thus, the patient's functioning in sensorimotor, perceptual, and cognitive areas is addressed as well as his overall functioning in daily living skills. Presence of dysfunction in these areas warrants further assessment of individual sensory systems including the vestibular, tactile, proprioceptive, kinesthetic, visual, auditory, gustatory, and olfactory systems. Dysfunction of these sensory systems is believed to contribute to the patient's overall sensory system dysfunction [7,49]. Standardized instruments, interviews, and observations are used for both screening and evaluation [49,71].

3. *Model of human occupation.* The purpose of assessment is to determine the degree of the patient's overall system organization. It is believed that the patient is an open system in which the state of his internal organization, external environment, or both determines how the system (patient) will function [57,59,83]. The patient's internal organization (throughput) is determined by assessing three subsystems (volition, habituation, performance) and their inter-relationships.

Presence of dysfunction in these three subsystems warrants further assessment of the components of each to determine the nature and extent of the patient's occupational dysfunction [57]. The fit between the patient and his environment and the fit between the patient's environmental demands and his opportunities are evaluated [9]. Standardized instruments, history taking, and clinical observations are used for screening and evaluation [10,57].

4. *Cognitive disabilities.* The purpose of assessment is to identify the extent of the patient's cognitive limitation and the degree to which it interferes with his performance of routine tasks [2]. It is postulated that psychiatric illness frequently results in residual cognitive disabilities that impair the patient's ability to function in his everyday life [1,2]. Presence of a cognitive deficiency warrants further assessment of the patient's routine task performance and application of activity analysis to these tasks. The focus of treatment is to facilitate the patient's best performance through environmental compensations or to structure the task so he is able to complete it successfully [1,2]. Standardized instruments are used to identify the patient's current cognitive level. History taking and observations are used in both screening and evaluation [2].

Your Turn

Not all areas included in the domain of concern are relevant to each frame of reference. In addition, each frame of reference organizes areas in the domain of concern in a different manner. This exercise provides a format to synthesize information about each frame of reference. You may find that you are unable to complete all the items at this time. Use these items as a guide for gathering additional information. References are provided at the end of the chapter for additional reading in each frame of reference.

For each area listed below, circle the code for the frame(s) of reference that addresses it in some manner and illustrate with an example. (Key: FP = functional performance, SI = sensory integration, HO = model of human occupation, CD = cognitive disabilities.)

1. Living situation and responsibilities:

   FP

   SI

   HO

   CD

2. Self-care/personal hygiene:

   FP

   SI

HO

CD

3. Homemaking:

FP

SI

HO

CD

4. Work:

FP

SI

HO

CD

5. Play and leisure:

FP

SI

HO

CD

6. Self-esteem and self-concept:

FP

SI

HO

CD

7. Situational coping

FP

SI

HO

CD

8. Self-expression and self-control:

FP

SI

HO

CD

9. Cognitive functioning:

FP

SI

HO

CD

10. Neuromuscular functioning:

FP

SI

HO

CD

11. Sensory integration:

    FP

    SI

    HO

    CD

12. Interpersonal relationships:

    FP

    SI

    HO

    CD

13. Environmental constraints and resources:

    FP

    SI

    HO

    CD

Summary
This section examined O.T.'s domain of concern in psychiatry and discussed the relationship of O.T. frames of reference to the assessment process. These frames of reference "are not recipes; they provide guidelines for practice only" [79].

By a man's finger-nails, by his coat-sleeve, by his boots, by his trouser-knees, by the callouses of his forefinger and thumb, by his expression, by his shirt-cuffs; by each of these things a man's calling is plainly revealed. That all united should fail to enlighten the competent inquirer, in any case, is almost inconceivable.

Sir Arthur Conan Doyle's Sherlock Holmes

The screening process involves identifying a patient who needs O.T., obtaining a referral, and collecting a data base. At that point, you analyze the data and make one of two decisions: you need more information about specific areas of functioning and thus proceed to the evaluation step, or you have enough information to identify problems.

Referrals

Each facility specifies procedures for identifying patients who need O.T. services. For example, patients may be identified by other health-care professionals and referred to O.T., or you may need to generate your own referrals by seeking out appropriate patients and requesting a referral. Attending staff meetings and reviewing patient's charts should give you enough information to initiate an appropriate referral. The days of "everyone can benefit from a little O.T." and "refer him to O.T., and I'll decide what to do next" are almost over. Realistically, there are limits to your ability to help every patient; not everyone can benefit from O.T. services. Unfortunately, no adequate guideline currently exists to determine which patients are appropriate referrals. Even if an occupational therapist believed that O.T. would benefit a patient, his services may not be reimbursable and therefore not sanctioned by the treatment facility. Determining who receives what kind of O.T. services is a complex decision based, in part, on the philosophy of the treatment institution, the frame(s) of reference used in O.T., and economic realities. Accountability for providing needed and effective services begins with selecting appropriate patients for O.T.

Most treatment facilities require some type of written referral for O.T. Although many regulatory and reimbursement agencies require the referral to be signed by a physician, some will accept those signed by other professionals. Patients can be referred under a blanket referral—that is, everyone in a given treatment program is referred to O.T. automatically—or they may be referred on a case-by-case basis. Receipt of a referral needs to be documented in the patient's chart. If you are able to screen the patient right away, the referral can be acknowledged as part of the initial note. However, if the screening is delayed for any reason (such as the patient's inability to cooperate because of intrusive symptoms, unavailability because of numerous other appointments, or refusal to attend O.T.), the referral must be documented in a separate note. See Chap. 4 for additional information on writing referral notes.

Frequently the stated reason for referral to O.T. is "to evaluate and treat." While that allows the occupational therapist the freedom and flexibility to provide whatever O.T. services he chooses, some regulatory agencies are starting to require a more specific reason for referral to O.T. Too much specificity, however, can create problems. Most occupational therapists have a favorite story about inappropriate referrals (for example, "to evaluate and motivate," or "to entertain the patient"). Because the referral is a legal document, you are obligated either to carry out what is requested on the referral or to state why it will not be done. To save yourself the time needed to respond to inappropriate referrals and yet ensure that you receive referrals when you need them, take a proactive stance. Make sure the wording reflects the services you wish to deliver, and present the referral to the source for a signature. Attend rounds and staff meetings regarding patients, and speak up about what O.T. can offer the patients discussed. Increasing your visibility and develop-

Fig. 2-1. A checklist for handling referrals.

Is a referral necessary to deliver O.T. services?

Who is the source of referrals? (specific names help the most)

What is the process for receiving referrals?

Where are the referrals put?

Who processes the doctor's orders?

How do you bring the need for the referral to the doctor's attention?

Is the process usually expedient?

Is there any way to speed up the process if there are delays?

Within what time frame do you need to respond to a referral?

How are weekend referrals handled?

Where is the note written in the chart?

What is the suggested format for responding to referral notes?

ing clear criteria for referral are effective strategies to increase the number of appropriate referrals to O.T. [84]. The specific wording of referrals varies with each frame of reference. Possibilities might include: to assess functional status of self-maintenance and leisure, to treat as indicted, to assess patient's sensory integrative functioning, to assess organization of patient's occupational functioning, or to monitor patient's functional abilities to assist in titration of medication [1,2,10,27,37,49,57,71, 79]. By preparing the referral yourself, you not only expedite the process, but you also educate the rest of the staff about the services you provide.

Identifying patients and responding to referrals may seem like an unimportant part of your job. In most places, however, a referral is needed to give you access to the patient. Without one, you generally cannot provide O.T. or be reimbursed for your services. Delays in obtaining referrals delay needed treatment and cost the O.T. department money. Responding to inappropriate referral wastes time that could be better spent working with patients. Although it is not glamorous, efficient handling of referrals facilitates the rest of your work. A guide to help you orient yourself to your facility's procedures is suggested in Fig. 2-1.

Your Turn
Using the principles of each frame of reference, prepare the wording for an appropriate O.T. referral.

Functional performance:

Sensory integration:

Model of human occupation:

Cognitive disabilities:

Establishing a Data Base

Once the patient has been identified and you have received a referral, the next step is to collect a data base. Ideally, the data base contains a chart review, an interview, and a performance measure. The chart review yields information about your patient's history, diagnosis, and reasons for seeking treatment. The interview reveals your patient's perspective on his disorder and his goals for treatment, and the performance measure indicates his ability to do or perform specific tasks. The data base would thus provide a rough indication of your patient's history, his awareness of his disorder, his treatment goals, and his ability to perform a given task. When these steps are completed, it is time to analyze the data and decide if you need additional information. If so, proceed with the evaluation; if not, identify areas of problems and strengths.

Chart Review

Should you read the patient's chart before meeting him? The argument that you might be biased by the information in the chart is contrasted with the arguments that you risk wasting your time as well as your patient's time, money, and goodwill by asking him the same questions everyone else has already asked and by needlessly duplicating services. You can use the first contact with your patient as an opportunity to engage his cooperation and build rapport (remember the preparing actions of Chap. 1?); however, you need to have a specific idea of what O.T. can offer him. Completing the chart review prior to meeting your patient can help you form a pre-assessment image [92, p. 605] that you can share with him during the interview. This image is a preliminary hypothesis of the patient's problems and is subject to revision and refinement as you gather more information. For these and the safety reasons mentioned in the "Precautions" section (p. 55), completing the chart review is recommended as the first step in collecting a data base.

The purpose of reading the patient's chart is to obtain enough information for you to make a preliminary identification of problems amenable to O.T. treatment, to select a frame of reference, to define a focus for the interview, and to choose a performance measure. You need to limit the information you record, as some patients have extensive documentation that could take hours to wade through. What is important for you to know at this point? A format for organization of the chart information is suggested in Fig. 2-2.

DIAGNOSIS

Your patient's diagnosis and reasons for seeking treatment can give you an idea of his symptoms and the course of his disorder. Although disagreement exists among occupational therapists about the usefulness of a psychiatric diagnosis, most third-party payers require a record of the patient's diagnosis in the O.T. documentation

```
Name:                          Date:

Physician:                     Diagnosis:

Medications:                   Precautions:

Presenting Problems:           Axis V:

Mental Status:

History of Present Illness:

Other:
```

Adapted from: Allen, C. *Occupational Therapy for Psychiatric Diseases: Measurement and Management of Cognitive Disabilities.* Boston: Little, Brown, 1985. P. 107.

for reimbursement purposes. Pragmatically, the diagnosis is usually required; conceptually, it can be used as indicated by each frame of reference. Diagnoses following the DMS III format have five axes [5]. It is assumed that you are familiar with both this format and the major diagnoses.

PRESENTING PROBLEMS

The patient's reasons for seeking treatment, or the presenting problems, are rarely just the diagnosis. For instance, not all people with schizophrenia or depression are in some type of treatment program, nor do they need to be. Usually the presenting problems are difficulties associated with or resulting from the disorder, such as danger to self or others or inability to care for self. Sometimes, the reason for treatment is to determine the diagnosis and rule out all other possibilities. Initial impressions are recorded by the physician as a working diagnosis that is subject to change or verification.

MEDICATIONS

Note the names, amounts, and starting dates of medications your patient is receiving. This information, added to your knowledge of the psychiatric disorder, helps you determine the appropriate type and timing of assessment. For example, if a patient diagnosed with bipolar illness, acute manic phase, was referred to O.T., you would anticipate that some of his symptoms would include increased activity levels, increased amount of speech, pressure of speech, flight of ideas, racing thoughts, and distractibility [5]. Assuming he was just started on lithium carbonate, you can also anticipate that it will take a week or more for his condition to stabilize. Even if you suspect that the patient exhibits difficulties in his ability to work, assessment of a skill when his symptoms are uncontrolled would likely reflect his disorder rather than his actual performance abilities. Not only would you waste time and money collecting useless information, but you also might be misled into thinking you needed to treat the problem at this time. Some problems self-correct when the patient's symptoms are controlled; thus assessments need to be timed appropriately. Many medications have side effects that you need to consider. Postural hypotension, blurry vision, fatigue, restlessness, tremor, and dry mouth are common. Some medications necessitate dietary restrictions, and noncompliance results in serious medical emergencies [102]. Awareness of these side effects is paramount for appropriate and humane treatment.

PRECAUTIONS

For safety reasons, you need to note whether the patient is on suicidal, homicidal, elopement, or fire precautions, as these have a direct effect on when and where you can see the patient and on the type of activity you can use. Each facility delineates procedures to handle these situations, and you should become familiar with them immediately.

MENTAL STATUS EXAM

A current determination of mental status, usually done by the psychiatrist or resident, will help you focus the interview and choose an appropriate performance measure. For example, if the patient is oriented times two (to person and place but not time), confused, and exhibits a short attention span, you can anticipate that the interview will need to be short and use closed questions. Depending on the severity of the symptoms, you may need to delay the interview until the patient is able to cooperate. You would also anticipate that the most successful performance measure would be one that is possible to complete in a short time.

HISTORY OF PRESENT ILLNESS

Finally, a brief history of the patient's illness, including previous hospitalizations, helps you predict his future level of functioning and set realistic treatment goals. Note whether DSM III axis V of the diagnosis is completed [5]. If not, identify the patient's highest level of functioning in the past year. (See Allen's refinement of the axis V criteria for additional information [2, p. 124].

Selecting a Frame of Reference

Selecting a frame of reference is the next step in the screening process. You can construct an outline for additional investigation by linking the principles of the frame of reference with your preassessment image of the patient [92]. As discussed earlier (p. 44), each frame of reference selects areas from our domain of concern to assess and identifies behaviors that indicate function and dysfunction in these areas [79]. To date, no clinically tested guideline exists to indicate when to use which frame of reference—leaving personal preference and belief as the basis of your choice [1]. Conceptual work has begun to identify groups of patients appropriate for particular frames of reference. For example, chronic process schizophrenics and developmentally disabled patients are suggested as appropriate for the sensory integration frame of reference [61], those with cognitive disabilities as appropriate for the cognitive disabilities frame of reference [2], and those with occupational dysfunction as appropriate for the model of human occupation [10]. Clinical outcome studies are needed to document the effectiveness of particular approaches with particular patient problems and diagnoses. You not only need to know which problems you can help, but you also need to know the best way to bring about the desired changes. Until these clinically tested guidelines become available, selection of the frame of reference can be based, in part, on the following logistical criteria.

EXPECTED LENGTH OF TREATMENT

Each type of treatment facility, whether it is an acute inpatient unit or a day care, outpatient, or residential treatment facility, has an expressed mission for service that affects your delivery of services. Failure to take this mission into account leads to inadequate treatment and frustration for both you and your patient. For example, acute inpatient units frequently attempt to limit the patient's length of stay to two weeks or less [103]. The treatment focuses on managing acute symptoms and discharging the patient as soon as he is medically stable. Obviously, this short length of stay limits the type of assessment and treatment you can expect to accomplish. Neglecting this reality can leave you planning unrealistic goals for assessment and treatment: work gets started, but not finished, and the patient leaves without feeling that O.T. did him much good. Possibly it did not. Some frames of reference imply a lengthy course of treatment, which would be futile to attempt in a short-term setting [88]. To prevent a needless exercise in frustration tolerance for both you and your patient, try not to undertake something that you cannot reasonably expect to finish.

FACILITY'S FRAME OF REFERENCE
There will be a general psychologic frame of reference that is used by most of the staff. It might be eclectic, or it might be limited to one particular approach (e.g., behavioral, biologic, analytic, humanistic, or cognitive). If you decide to use an O.T. frame of reference that is not complementary to the rest of the staff's approach, you will have several problems. The information you generate may not seem valuable to the rest of the staff, you will need to undertake major re-education of the staff about the frame of reference you are using and what it means, and in some cases you may lose referrals for patients if the doctor or referral source disagrees with what you are proposing to do. This discussion is not meant to discourage you from thinking things through on your own and deciding on your best approach. It just points out the difficulties you might encounter so you can be prepared.

RESOURCES AVAILABLE
If you wish to use a frame of reference that is not generally used by the occupational therapists at your facility, do you have the time, space, supplies, and support needed to implement it? Will the services you intend to provide be reimbursed? Being able to make a change in your treatment facility's program is exciting and challenging. Yet lack of careful advance planning can thwart your well-intended efforts. In addition to good planning, tact and diplomacy are essential weapons in effecting change. Fidler presents helpful strategies for program planning and effecting change in her text, *Design of Rehabilitation Services in Psychiatric Hospital Settings* [34].

Interview
Almost everyone working in psychiatry interviews patients; thus your interview must be focused to prevent needless duplication of services. The purpose of this screening interview is to collect information and establish rapport with the patient. The topics you discuss will reflect O.T.'s domain of concern as conceived by the frame of reference you have selected. Although some are more articulated than others, each frame of reference provides guidelines for the content and format of the screening interview. Recall from Chap. 1 that interviews can be structured, semistructured, or unstructured. The following information is a summary of suggested interview content and format for each frame of reference. It is for comparison purposes only; additional study of the frames of reference is required before you conduct your interview. Space has been left to encourage you to add to the list as you continue your studies.

1. *Content.* Explore the patient's activity history, family patterns that shaped attitudes and values, current activity pattern, role performance at work and play, self-maintenance roles, and environmental resources/barriers [27,33,34,36].

   Notes:

2. *Format.* Semistructured; the Lifestyle Performance Profile Occupational History and the Role Activity Performance Scale are suggested [33,41].

   Notes:

SENSORY INTEGRATION

1. *Content.* Review childhood development, academic, and medical histories. Look for incidences of neurologic disorders in the family, delayed development, neurologic soft signs, or childhood hyperactivity [41,49,62].

   Notes:

2. *Format:* Structured; Self-Reported Childhood History section of the Schroeder, Block, and Campbell (SBC) evaluation is suggested [96].

   Notes:

MODEL OF HUMAN OCCUPATION

1. *Content.* Explore the patient's organization of volition, habituation, and performance subsystems. Explore environmental press, opportunities, and fit. Topics may include values, personal causation, interests, roles, habits, performance skills, and environmental interaction patterns [9,10,60,107].

   Notes:

2. *Format.* Semistructured; Occupational Therapy Functional Screening Tool [107], Occupational Role History [38], and Occupational Case Analysis [54] are suggested.

   Notes:

COGNITIVE DISABILITIES

1. *Content.* Explore patient's routine task behavior. Topics covered may include education, work, hospitalization history, nature of patient's environment out-

side the treatment setting, social supports available, recent typical day, goals, and self-assessment of strengths and limitations [2].

Notes:

2. *Format.* Semistructured; Allen's Interview of Routine Task Behavior is suggested [2].

Notes:

Performance Measure

So far your data base consists of information you gathered from the chart review and interview. The final step of the screening process is to assess your patient's actual performance abilities in a given area. Psychiatric disorders often create problems in the patient's ability to perform in some way [2,10,36,60,61,63,79,95]. A vast discrepancy often exists between the patient's verbal abilities and his ability actually to perform [36,79]. Because one of O.T.s concerns is the patient's ability to perform activities that he needs and wants to do in his life [2,10,27,36,63], a global measure of his performance is essential. Basing your treatment on the patient's verbal self-reports alone is not adequate. Psychiatric disorders often create distorted concepts of one's actual performance abilities. Engaging your patient's cooperation in completing a performance measure must be handled carefully. For some patients, the performance measure requires them to do the very thing that is extremely difficult for them to do: perform in some way. Consequently, it brings them face to face with their limitations. This can be uncomfortable, frustrating, and demoralizing for the patient. Good rapport and the sensitivity to continue the performance measure only as long as needed to get an idea of your patient's functioning will minimize his discomfort. Performance measures are used in the screening process to detect global dysfunction in performance abilities. Presence of dysfunction in some area warrants indepth evaluation of that area. (See the section on "Evaluation," p. 72, for further information about performance measures.) As with interviews, each frame of reference provides guidelines for the content and format of performance measures. The following information is summarized for comparison purposes only. Additional study of the frames of reference is required before selecting a performance measure.

FUNCTIONAL PERFORMANCE

1. *Content.* Assess patient's performance of work, self-maintenance, and leisure roles. The balance of these roles is also examined. Task, interpersonal, and general behaviors may be assessed [27,33,79].

Notes:

2. *Format.* No specific performance measure for screening is identified; clinical observations of the patient's task behavior are used. Selected evaluation instruments may be useful in some situations, especially those that require actual per-

formance of the skills, such as the Scorable Self-Care Evaluation (SSCE) [25] or the Kohlman Evaluation of Living Skills (KELS) [75].

Notes:

SENSORY INTEGRATION

1. *Content.* Assess the patient's sensory system functioning, gross and fine motor development, neurophysiologic maturity, attention, behavior, perception, and daily living skills [49,71,96,105].

   Notes:

2. *Format.* No specific screening tool is identified; use of standardized instruments and clinical observations is recommended [49]. Selected evaluation instruments may be useful in some situations.

   Notes:

MODEL OF HUMAN OCCUPATION

1. *Content.* Assessment of the performance subsystem including motor, process, and communication/interpersonal skills [57].

   Notes:

2. *Format.* No specific performance-screening measure of the performance sub-system is identified; clinical observations are used. Selected evaluation instruments such as the Bay Area Functional Performance Evaluation (BaFPE) [17] or the Comprehensive Occupational Therapy Evaluation (COTE) [21] may be useful in some situations.

   Notes:

COGNITIVE DISABILITIES

1. *Content.* Make an initial determination of the patient's cognitive level [1,2].

   Notes:

2. *Format.* Observation plus Allen Cognitive Level Test (ACL) and the Lower Cognitive Level Test (LCL) are recommended [1,2].

   Notes:

Preliminary Data Synthesis

Assuming data collection has proceeded as described, you have lots of information to synthesize. Frequently, however, the data collection process does not follow this sequence. At times, your patient's symptoms may prevent him from cooperating in a reliable self-report, and the interview must be delayed. If for some reason the performance measure is given first, you will not have had the opportunity provided by the interview to build rapport. In that case, the preparing and attending actions of Chap. 1 become especially useful in building rapport rapidly and engaging your patient's cooperation in attempting the performance measure. Although chart review is a good first step, it does not yield sufficient information alone to plan treatment. If both the interview and the performance measure are delayed, defer treatment planning and implementation until they can be completed. The order and depth of the screening reflect each patient's needs; yet the entire screening process is needed to provide adequate data for treatment planning.

By this point in your professional education, you have surely been introduced to the concept: evaluate before you treat. Nonetheless, the realities of clinical practice, such as large case loads, busy schedules, and limited resources, create pressure to treat the patient as soon as possible. In some settings, especially acute inpatient facilities, extensive assessment is not possible. Rather than abandoning or short-changing the assessment in order to start treatment quickly, we need to refine our current screening and evaluation procedures for speed and efficiency and to develop new screening instruments.

Finally, determine whether you have enough information at this point to proceed with treatment planning. Did you get a rough idea of your patient's functioning in all the areas specified by your frame of reference? Were there areas that warranted further evaluation? Can initial problems be identified and treatment begun even if you do not have a complete data base? To determine whether you have enough information, read the section on "Problem Identification" (p. 88) and try the exercises. If you are able to complete this step successfully, you can proceed with setting goals, objectives, and methods (Chap. 3). Do not forget to read the section on "Evaluation" (p. 64), even if you are not using it at this moment. If you are not able to identify problems with your current amount of information, identify the specific areas of functioning that need further evaluation, and proceed with the next step: evaluation. You will have to settle for some degree of incomplete information. As stated in the Laundry List of Eternal Truths, "All important decisions must be made on the basis of insufficient data" [85]. You may not have all the information you would like, but determining the cutoff point will become easier with your increased understanding of psychiatric disorders, the frames of reference, and clinical experience.

Your Turn

The following case study provides an opportunity for you to apply what you just learned about collecting a data base. Given the following information, complete the chart review form, select a frame of reference, and identify the content and format for both the interview and performance measures.

Background Data

TREATMENT FACILITY

The facility is a 24-bed acute inpatient unit in a general hospital where the average length of stay is 10 to 14 days. The unit heavily emphasizes medical intervention and short intensive therapy aimed at controlling or eliminating the patient's symptoms and connecting the patient with community resources for continued therapy, if required.

OCCUPATIONAL THERAPY DEPARTMENT

One full-time and one part-time Occupational Therapist, Registered (O.T.R.) work in this unit. The O.T. department is eclectic in its use of frames of reference.

PATIENT INFORMATION

Psychiatrist's Admission Note Date: February 8. Patient (Susan) is a 45-year-old divorced white female who was first seen January 31 when brought by younger brother to office. Reported recent flight from job as music coordinator at regional school district in neighboring state. Susan was hired for a new job last October. The hiring was a political issue and was contested. Partly through the pressure of friends, Susan was selected for the job. She recently graduated from college with a degree in education, spent her first year teaching junior high music classes, and then was hired for this current job. As the semester progressed, Susan felt more and more pressure and was less able to supervise teachers with more experience than she. She was also feeling the loss of her second son, who had moved away from home to attend college. Her other son lives at some distance. Susan was divorced 13 years ago; her exhusband died 3 years ago. His death was difficult for Susan, as he had apparently been a support. Susan had a long-standing relationship with a man and was disappointed that this relationship had not led to marriage. This is the first psychiatric hospitalization. Susan denies other episodes of depression. No family history of depression can be ascertained. Family consists of two sisters and one brother; Susan is the oldest. Parents live locally, and Susan alternates staying with them and with her younger brother. She left her job and home precipitously, left a note for her male friend, and drove herself to her parents' home (7-hour drive) "crying all the way."

On evaluation of mental status patient gave the following impression: alert, somewhat reticent to talk (but would respond to direct questions), slowed motorically, speech fluent, mood depressed. Affect showed appropriateness (i.e., was able to smile at humorous remarks, but smile seemed forced). Reported feeling guilty, trapped, but not hopeless. Has had suicidal thought involving driving car into the lake; no attempt. Sleep is characterized by frequent awakening. Reported recent weight loss of 14 pounds. Patient states that she is not eating to "punish herself." Feels a burden to her relatives.

Diagnosis
1. Major depressive episode
2. Rule out situational depression, dysthymia

Treatment
1. Nortriptyline HCl (Pamelor) 25 mg on 2/8 (start 50 mg on 2/10)
2. Alprazolam (XANAX) 0.25 mg b.i.d.
3. Occupational therapy
4. Groups on unit as tolerated

Nursing Admission Note. This 45-year-old divorced woman was admitted by Dr. James. Susan is the mother of two sons: Albert, 23, who works out of state, and Michael, 18, who attends college where Susan lives. Susan recently finished her bachelor's degree in music education and taught for 1 year. Last October she took over as music coordinator in a 20-school system where she was expected to supervise other music teachers and teach in as many elementary schools as she could. She found this job stressful. Her anxiety increased; she ate very little and was not able to sleep. About 2 weeks ago she left her job and came to stay with her parents in town. Six years ago she worked in a sheltered workshop with developmentally disabled adults. When she was promoted, she became anxious and walked off the job. Three years ago her exhusband died unexpectedly. He had remarried 3 weeks before his death; she was not aware of this until his funeral. She states she has not adequately grieved this loss. She reports that recently she has had a poor relationship with her son Michael. She feels rejected by him. He is dating a woman Susan does not like. Susan states that she is suffering from "empty nest syndrome." Another recent stress is a long-standing relationship with a man that "didn't go anywhere." She attempted to sell her house so she could live with her older son, but the house did not sell. She has had fleeting thoughts of suicide. Two weeks ago she had a biopsy of a lump in her breast, which was benign. Admission weight of 106 was down from normal 127.

Vital signs
1. Temperature: 97.2; Pulse: 76; Respirations: 18
2. Blood pressure: 116/80
3. Height: 5'5"
4. Weight: 106 lb

Reason for hospitalization/chief complaint/symptoms: Has been depressed over multiple losses; latest is job.
Other illnesses: Biopsy of right breast lump 2 weeks ago; nonmalignant.
Vision: Within normal limits.
Hearing: Within normal limits.
Speech: Within normal limits.
Cardiac: Denies problems.
Peripheral vascular: Denies problems; routine physical scheduled 2/9.
Respiratory: Denies problems.
Neurologic: Denies problems.
Musculoskeletal: Denies problems.
Reproductive: Hysterectomy 5 years ago.
Gastrointestinal: Poor eating habits, causing constipation.
Urinary: Denies problems.

Chart Review
Using the information from Susan's chart, complete the chart review. Note any terminology or medication with which you are unfamiliar so you can look it up later.

Name: Date:

Physician: Diagnosis:

Medications: Precautions:

Presenting problems:

Mental status:

History of present illness:

Additional:

Identifying Frame of Reference
Based on the information collected so far and the background data about the treatment facility, which frame of reference would you use?

Basis for selection:

Interview
Based on your knowledge of this patient and the constructs of the frame of reference you selected, identify the format and content of the screening interview.

1. *Format* (Specify the name, if applicable):

2. *Content* (Identify the topics you would address. If the format you selected is not standardized, write a primary question to introduce each topic.):

Performance Measure
Finally, select the format and content of the performance measure you would use.

1. *Format* (Specify the name, if applicable):

2. *Content* (Specify the areas included):

You have completed as much of the screening process as possible without a patient. Next you would conduct the interview and performance measure and decide whether you need more information (evaluation) or whether you should proceed directly to problem identification.

Summary
This selection introduced screening as the first step in the assessment process. Screening consists of referral, chart review, interview, and performance measure. The next step of the assessment process is evaluation, and it includes both principles of measurement and types of evaluation instruments.

Evaluation

[The] first requirement is [to] know the rules thoroughly so they can be applied to any situation. Second is to follow the rules implicitly, but objectively use them to best [sic] of your ability. Third is a tremendous amount of good judgment to anticipate the variables. And fourth, a small amount of good luck.

Pat Royce
The Sailor's Bible

For many years, informal observations and nonstandardized rating scales served as the primary evaluation tools in psychiatric O.T. [81]. Development of standardized psychiatric O.T. instruments began in the 1970s and continues today—and just in time. The rapid changes in the treatment of psychiatric disorders mandate that we use efficient and cost-effective means of patient evaluation. In some settings, time and financial constraints prohibit extensive, lengthy evaluation. Unless the patient is evaluated rapidly, the opportunity to provide needed treatment is missed. "Today's therapist must enter the evaluation process well prepared, knowing beforehand what questions to ask and how to get the best answers regardless of the instruments being used [19, p. 28]. All occupational therapists working in psychiatry are experiencing an increased demand for demonstrated evidence that the patient needed and benefited from O.T. services. Standardized instruments are part of the arsenal of weapons we need to repond to these challenges.

At this point in the assessment process, you have completed the screening of your patient, and you have an idea of the areas that need further evaluation. Selection of an evaluation instrument begins with understanding the principles of measurement.

Principles of Measurement

Does it matter if an instrument is not standardized? Yes and no. The process of standardization helps to minimize the amount of error in your results that is due to the instrument itself. Standardized instruments give us some degree of confidence that the patient's rating reflects his actual performance, *not* the way the instrument was developed, administered, scored, or interpreted. Nonstandardized instruments, although useful in some respects, must be interpreted with considerable caution because we have no way of knowing whether the rating accurately represents the patient's performance or how much of the rating reflects measurement error. The more we know about an instrument's psychometric properties, the more appropriately we can use it and interpret the results. A standardized instrument includes a description of its purpose, an administration and scoring protocol, and established norms, reliability, and validity [16].

Administration and Scoring Protocol

ADMINISTRATION PROTOCOL

Specifying a protocol for administering the instrument enables any therapist to give it in the same manner [16]. The protocol usually includes the type of evaluation environment, the materials needed, the order in which the materials or items are presented, and the exact wording of the directions you would give to the patient. Does it really matter if the administration protocol is followed exactly? Suppose you forgot to get all the materials out of the cupboard before you began the evaluation (not recommended as part of the administration protocol). Would getting up to retrieve the materials during the evaluation session have a significant effect? Maybe not, but the problem is that you cannot determine just how much of an effect it would have. Your actions could be interpreted by your patient as disinterest, incompetence, or distracting. Because you would not be able to tell how much of an effect the interruption had on your patient's performance, you would have invalidated his rating. Minor variations in protocol can have a larger effect than you might at first think.

Allen reports that a false high rating on the ACL test can occur if the therapist merely adds the words "stop and think" to the directions [2]. If an instrument does not have an administration protocol, each therapist using it will administer it in a different manner and will probably obtain different results, thus making comparison of the results difficult. In summary, the administration protocol helps eliminate the manner in which the instrument is given as a contributing source of error in the patient's rating. Unless you follow the protocol exactly, you will not be able to determine if your patient's rating accurately reflects his performance or if it is a false rating created, in part, by the way you administered the instrument.

SCORING PROTOCOL

The scoring protocol identifies all possible ratings and the criteria for determining these ratings. Its purpose is to produce the same rating for the same performance regardless of who completes the rating, thus increasing consistency of ratings from one therapist to another. Specific directions and rating keys that allow as little room as possible for disagreement among raters will improve the rating's objectivity and consistency [106].

Norms

Normative data describe the range of ratings on the instrument for a specific population. Norms can be collected for different populations, such as age groups, diagnostic categories, or genders [18]. Norms are usually stated as measures of central tendency (i.e., mean and standard deviation), and they are useful for putting your patient's rating on the instrument into some context. For instance, norms can identify how your patient's rating compares to ratings obtained by other patients with similar characteristics (age, gender, diagnosis) or to those of a "normal" population. The more closely your patient can be matched to the normed population in demographic characteristics, the more confidence you can place in the comparison. Use of normative data for dissimilar populations results in an inaccurate interpretation of the results. For instance, the Southern California Sensory Integration Tests (SCSIT) have norms for children [6]. If these tests are used with adults to indicate suspected sensory integrative dysfunction, the results must be viewed with extreme caution. Comparing adult performance to that of children implies that their performance on the SCSIT is comparable. Although efforts are being made to collect data about adult performance on the SCSIT [52,86,87], at this writing we still do not have enough information to make an accurate interpretation of impaired adult performance. Relating an adult's performance to children's norms (for example, patient scored in the 75th percentile for an 8-year-old) implies that his performance is poor for an adult. We just do not know yet if this is the case.

In summary, norms provide a context for interpreting the patient's ratings to determine his degree of function and dysfunction as compared with a "normal" population, other patients, or both.

Reliability

Considered by some to be the most important aspect of standardization, reliability refers to the consistency and stability of the instrument. If an instrument is reliable, you can expect it to produce similar results if used with the same patient at two different times (test-retest reliability) or if used and scored by two different observers (interobserver or inter-rater reliability) [16].

What makes the reliability of an instrument so important? An instrument with high reliability usually indicates that the problems it measures are well enough defined that the instrument identifies them in the same person more than once. Additionally, the problem was well enough defined that, unlike the six blind men describing an elephant, two raters looking at the same thing generally agree on what they see. Reliability, however, does not mean the same thing as accuracy. An instrument can be reliable, but inaccurate. Suppose you weighed yourself on your bathroom scale every week, and your scale consistently read the same weight. Your weight really stayed the same (you double-checked it at the gym to make sure), so you can say that your bathroom scale was reliable. You might not be happy about the weight it registered, but you would have to admit it was reliable. If you gained or lost weight but your scale continued to register the same weight as before, the scale would still be reliable (since the readings were consistent), but it certainly would not be accurate.

Test-retest reliability indicates that the instrument is stable over a period of time. That is, it identifies the same problems in the same person over time with a greater than chance probability. If the instrument has high test-retest reliability, you can be reasonably confident that changes in your patient's rating on a second administration of the instrument reflect actual changes in his performance rather than measurement errors. Adequate test-retest reliability is a prerequisite if you plan to use the same instrument for evaluation and re-evaluation of the patient to determine his treatment outcome [8]. Without established test-retest reliability of the instrument, you would not be able to tell whether the changes in your patient's rating reflected changes caused by the treatment or changes caused by instability of the instrument.

Interobserver reliability refers to the degree to which two observers agree with each other in the observing, scoring, and judging of the same phenomenon [4]. As mentioned previously, high interobserver reliability is a good indicator of the specificity of the items being evaluated. If interobserver reliability is high, you can have confidence that, if you follow the administration and scoring protocols, your rating of a patient's performance will be consistent with the way other therapists would rate the same performance.

Reliability is usually established during the development of the instrument. Test-retest reliability is determined by administering the same instrument, or a parallel form of the instrument, twice to the same person or group [14]. The timing between these trials is a critical factor in determining test-retest reliability. If the period is too short, the subject may recall answers from the first trial, sometimes referred to as the *practice effect* or *false positives* [17]. Conversely, if the interval is too long, the subject may have changed in some way. If the instrument reflects these changes, it appears to have low reliability [16]. Test-retest reliability studies of instruments therefore need to be timed to minimize the variable of unwanted changes in the test subjects. Three to five weeks between trials is common [17].

Interobserver reliability is established by comparing the ratings of two or more observers of the same subject. Frequently the subject is videotaped, and the observers view the tape and rate the subject's performance using the instrument. Ratings are compared to determine the amount of agreement between the raters [16].

Reliability is determined statistically and presented either as a correlation or a percentage of agreement. There is little practical difference between the two forms; both indicate the degree to which the two items compared (either the pretest–post-test or the two observers) relate. A perfect correlation of 1.0 (100%) means that the two items are identical; the subject would score exactly the same on the pretest and post-test, or both observers would rate the subject in exactly the same way. This is nearly impossible to achieve; thus a correlation of 0.80 or 80 percent is generally accepted as high reliability [14]. Some researchers suggest that a 0.70 (70%) correlation is adequate, but basically the higher the correlation, the more confidence you can place in the instrument's reliability. Remember, a high correlation does not imply cause and effect, but merely indicates a relationship between things. For example, a high correlation between alcohol consumption and low grades does not mean that the first caused the latter, only that the two are related in some way.

In summary, reliability indicates the instrument's stability. If test-retest reliability is high, you can be confident that the instrument is measuring the same patient performances on the second trial as it did on the first trial. Such an instrument would be appropriate to use to measure outcome of treatment through evaluation and re-evaluation. If the interobserver reliability is high, you can be confident that the patient performances and criteria for determining ratings are well enough defined that anyone using the instrument would rate behaviors in a similar way. This assures you that you are rating the patient in the way intended by the instrument's designers. In both instances, high reliability means you can count on the instrument to do the same thing trial after trial; however, it does not ensure the accuracy of what you are measuring.

Validity

Validity indicates the instrument's accuracy, or its ability to measure what it is supposed to measure. If you are not sure that the instrument really measures what it claims to measure, it is as useful to you as the broken bathroom scale. Validity cannot be established in the abstract; it is related to a specific purpose and population. Several types of validity can be determined: face, content, criterion, and construct.

FACE VALIDITY

Face validity globally represents how well the instrument appears to measure what it proposes to measure [22]. Face validity is determined by a subjective judgment, usually made by a panel of experts, that the instrument appears accurate. In general, face validity addresses the overall fit of the instrument with the target behaviors of the population it proposes to measure. So, "on the face of it," the instrument seems to fulfill its intended purpose.

CONTENT VALIDITY

Content validity represents how well the content of the instrument samples the topic under investigation. Content validity is often considered along with face validity. Whereas face validity is a global measure, content validity indicates the relevance and accuracy of each specific item on the instrument for its stated purpose and population. High content validity, also determined by experts, indicates that the topic is completely and accurately covered and can be adequately measured by the instrument under scrutiny. The instrument may also be pilot tested on a group of subjects similar to the target population to assist in developing content validity [14].

Although it may not be foremost on your mind, you are familiar with informal face and content validity. Think back to your last examination. When the test was first passed out, you probably scanned it to decide if the major topics covered reflected the material covered in class or if the professor had included some surprise questions. That was establishing face validity. As you took the test, you no doubt noticed how many of the questions related to each of the topics covered in class. You could tell which areas were covered in detail and which were barely addressed; especially if you were unprepared in some areas. You probably also made an assessment of how well the questions were written, if they were accurate, and if they were all relevant. You thus informally established content validity (we're assuming you are an expert in taking tests by now).

Because they depend on subjective judgments, face and content validity are not adequate, for most instruments, as the only forms of validity. Even though the judgments are made by experts, they are still subjective; other, more empirical forms of validity also must be established. In summary, face and content validity are expert "eyeballing" of the instrument to determine if the content really measures what the instrument claims to measure for the population it addresses.

CRITERION VALIDITY

Criterion validity is demonstrated by comparing the instrument to another measure with pre-established validity. The second measure is then used as a yardstick, or criterion, to validate the first. Why, you might ask, would you want to develop a new instrument if you already had another one that was valid and measured about the same thing? For several reasons: The new instrument might be easier to use, useful with a broader range of patients, or address a different aspect of the topic [16]. Criterion validity includes both concurrent and predictive validity. Both compare the instrument to another instrument, but at different times. This relationship between the two instruments is expressed as a correlation subjected to a test of significance. The higher the correlation, the better degree of criterion validity exists. Significance at the 0.05 level is acceptable; 0.01 is better [106].

Concurrent Validity. Concurrent validity is established by comparing the results of the instrument being developed with the results of another instrument (with established validity) that is given to the patient at about the same time, or concurrently [4,106]. A significant correlation of concurrent validity gives you confidence that the new instrument measures the target behaviors in a similar manner as the established measure. Thus, you can use the new instrument with some confidence of its accuracy.

Predictive Validity. Predictive validity is established by correlating the results of the instrument with another instrument (with established validity) given at a later date. If the correlation between the two is significant, the first instrument's scores could be said to predict the outcome of the second [4,43,106].

In summary, criterion validity indicates the instrument's accuracy through comparison with other established measures of the same target behaviors.

CONSTRUCT VALIDITY

Construct validity indicates the relationship of the instrument to a particular theory or frame of reference [106]. It is a measure of how well the instrument distinguishes among people (e.g., diagnostic categories, groups) based on theoretic predictions. Studies of construct validity essentially examine both the instrument and the frame of reference on which it is based. Establishing construct validity is a complex process. The construct to be tested is defined based on the principles of a frame of reference. "A construct is an ability, aptitude, trait, or characteristic that is hypothesized to explain some aspect of human behavior" [105, p. 338]. Hypotheses about how a patient who possesses either high or low degrees of this construct will perform on the instrument are identified [14]. Persons with high and low degrees of the construct are given the instrument, and their ratings are compared to the hypothesis to see how well the theory predicted their performance on the instrument. In other words, how much did the theoretic constructs account for the patient's performance on the instrument? Did the constructs accurately predict the patient's performance? If construct validity is established, we have confidence that the instrument can distinguish between persons based on the tested construct [106]. Constructs are complex phenomena, and one instrument or one observation is not sufficient to determine their existences. Construct validity studies normally use a number of instruments to assess a number of hypothesized predictions. For example, suppose one wanted to test a theoretic construct that high degrees of empathy are needed for effective occupational therapists. One hypothesis could be that O.T. students with high degrees of empathy would receive excellent ratings on their fieldwork and would score high on a hypothetical empathy scale. The other hypothesis then would be that O.T. students with low degrees of empathy would receive failing ratings on their fieldwork and would score low on the empathy scale. After all the data were collected, one could try to determine whether empathy was indeed related to fieldwork performance, and whether particular ratings on the empathy scale could predict a student's performance on their fieldwork. This example is somewhat simplistic; in actual practice the process of establishing construct validity is more complex and extensive.

In summary, the instrument is said to have construct validity if it shows a significant relationship between its construct and the hypothesized prediction or patients' scores on the instrument [14,106].

As a profession, O.T. is making progress in the standardization of instruments. The psychometric properties of some frequently used instruments in psychiatric O.T. are summarized in Table 2-1. These instruments are described further in the next section (pp. 73–87). Even though not completely standardized, our instruments can be used to guide and structure our observations if we keep their limitations in mind. The process of standardizing an instrument was described in some detail to impress on you that making up your own evaluation is not that simple. Nonstandardized instruments severely limit our ability to make definitive statements about the patient's functioning. Before doing it yourself, thoroughly check out all the O.T. instruments that already exist. Rather than starting from scratch, perhaps you can become involved in helping to standardize those that we already have and contribute to the development of our collective knowledge base.

Your Turn

Before using any instrument, you should get into the habit of reading the standardization data to learn about its psychometric properties and how the data were collected. Critical review of an instrument makes the principles discussed in this section more meaningful. Select an O.T. instrument to review, such as the Bay Area Functional Performance Evaluation (BaFPE) [17] or the Scorable Self Care Evaluation (SSCE) [22]. As you review the instrument, answer the following questions:

Protocols

1. Is there an administration protocol?

2. Is there a scoring protocol?

3. Were these protocols field tested with therapists other than the developers of the instrument?

Thoughts about the administration and scoring protocols:

Norms

4. Does the instrument have norms?

5. What groups were data collected on?

6. Are both normal and patient groups included?

Table 2-1. Summary of reported data on evaluation instrument's psychometric properties

Instrument	AP	SP	N	IR	TR	FV	CV	CCV	PV	CSV
Interviews										
Occupational role history	X	X		X						
Occupational case analysis	X	X		X		X	X			
Occupational functioning tool	X	X		X	X		X	X		
Role activity performance scale	X	X		X				X		
Adolescent role assessment	X	X								
Routine task history	X									
Self-Monitoring										
All instruments						X				
Self-report										
Activity configuration										
Self-directed search	X	X	X		X	X	X	X	X	X
Interest checklist					X					X
Role checklist	X				X	X	X			
Leisure satisfaction index	X			NA		X	X			
Life attitude profile	X	X	X	NA	X	X	X	X		
Rating										
Comprehensive O.T. evaluation		X		X						
Prevocational assessment of rehabilitation potential		X								X
Task										
Bay area functional performance evaluation	X	X	X	X			X	X		X
Scorable self-care evaluation	X	X	X	X	X					
Kohlman evaluation of living skills	X	X	X							
Allen cognitive level test	X	X		X			X	X	X	
Neuropsychologic										
SBC adult psychiatric integration evaluation	X	X		X						
Person symbol	X	X	X	X				X		
Projective										
Collage	X	X		X		X	X			X
B. H. Battery	X	X		X						

AP = administration protocol, SP = scoring protocol, N = norms, IR = interrater reliability, TR = test-retest reliability, FV = face validity, CV = content validity, CCV = concurrent validity, PV = predictive validity, CSV = construct validity, X = Reported data only; does not imply presence of the property in acceptable levels, NA = not available.

Thoughts about the normative data:

Reliability

7. Has the instrument established test-retest reliability?

8. If yes, what is the correlation?

9. How much time elapsed between the first and second administrations of the instrument in the test-retest studies?

10. Was that time appropriate?

11. What is your basis for that opinion?

12. Has the instrument established interobserver reliability?

13. If yes, what is the correlation?

14. How many observers were used?

15. Were the observers not the developers of the instrument?

16. Were the observers trained?

Thoughts about the reliability studies:

Validity

17. For what patient group is the instrument valid?

18. For what purpose is the instrument valid?

19. Has the instrument established face validity?

20. Has the instrument established content validity?

21. How were face and content validity established?

22. If a panel of experts were used, did it include therapists other than the developers of the instrument?

23. How were the times on the instrument selected?

24. Has the instrument established criterion validity?

25. If concurrent validity was established, what was the correlation and level of significance?

26. If concurrent validity, what other instruments were used?

27. What types of validity were established on the other instruments?

28. If predictive validity was established, what was the correlation and level of significance?

29. If predictive validity, what other instruments were used?

30. What types of validity were established on the other instruments?

31. Has the instrument established construct validity?

32. What hypotheses were tested?

33. What theory base or frame of reference was used?

Thoughts about the validity studies:

Overall impression of the instrument (include its strengths, limitations, and possible uses):

Evaluation Instruments

Occupational therapists working in psychiatry use a wide variety of instruments. Some were developed by occupational therapists, others were borrowed from other professions. In order to make an informed selection of an instrument, you need to know both the types of instruments available and their intended purposes. This section discusses several types: interviews, self-monitoring instruments, self-report instruments, behavior ratings, task evaluations, neurophysiologic instruments, and projective instruments.

Interviews

As you learned in the last section, the interview is an integral part of the screening process. It can also be used to obtain more specific information about a particular topic. Some interviews have scoring protocols that are used to rate and interpret the data obtained. As mentioned previously, interviews elicit a large amount of information in a relatively short time, and they yield information about the patient's perception of the topics addressed. The major disadvantage to interviews is that the patient must be able to provide a reliable self-report. Because they depend on the patient's viewpoint, interviews are subject to that person's biases and distortions. Of course, if the purpose of the interview is to identify the patient's viewpoint, then any biases represent his unique view and are not problematic. Conversely, if the purpose is to identify the patient's actual performance of a target behavior, then an interview, or any self-report instrument, will not be adequate as the only source of evaluation. Selected evaluation interview instruments are described in Fig. 2-3.

Self-Monitoring Instruments

Self-monitoring instruments are used by the patient to record the incidence of a problem as it occurs rather than in retrospect [8]. They rely on the patient learning to recognize that the problem has occurred and then promptly recording it. Patient compliance with this self-monitoring process is critical for collecting accurate and useful information. Self-monitoring instruments are most appropriately used to collect data about the patient's problems that cannot be directly observed by others [8,16]. Who can better monitor the occurrence of ruminating thoughts or feelings of anxiety than the person who has them? Self-monitoring instruments are individually created for each patient to record his perceptions, feelings, or thoughts about his problem. Like interviews, self-monitoring instruments require that the patient is able to cooperate and provide reliable data. Additionally, self-monitoring suffers

Fig. 2-3. Examples of interview instruments.

1. *The Occupational Role History* (ORH) was first developed by Moorhead [76] and revised by Florey and Michelman [38]. It was designed for use as a screening tool for short-term acutely ill adult psychiatric patients. Based on the model of human occupation, it collects information on role status and balance of leisure and role activities. Two occupational roles are included: worker/homemaker and student. The administration protocol provided allows addition and deletion of questions. Results are rated on a scale of 1 to 5, with 5 being "highly functional," in 11 component areas (values, personal causation, interests, internalized roles, habits, skills, intake, environment, feedback, output, and system trajectory [42]). Preliminary reliability studies are reported [42].

2. *Occupational Case Analysis* (OCA) was developed by Kaplan as a screening tool for short-term, acutely ill psychiatric patients in a hospital setting. Emphasis is on discharge planning [54]. Based on the model of human occupation, it yields information about each of 14 concepts of that model and includes questions on 10 primary topics (personal causation, values/goals, interests, internalized roles, habit patterns, skills, output, physical environment, social environment, and feedback). Results are rated on a scale of 1 to 5, with 5 as the most adaptive behavior. It also includes a rating of the patient's global functioning on four aspects of overall system functioning (dynamic, historic, contextual, system trajectory). There are scoring and administration protocols. Preliminary studies suggest inter-rater reliability as well as face and content validity. The instrument was revised after testing.

3. *The Occupational Functioning Tool* (OFT) was developed by Watts, Kielhofner, Bauer, Gregory, and Valentine as a screening tool for the institutionalized elderly [107]. Based on the model of human occupation, it yields information about six components (values, personal causation, interests, roles, habits, and skills). Results are rated on a scale of 1 to 5, with 1 as the most functional behavior. The administration protocol allows the addition and deletion of questions. There is a scoring protocol. Test-retest reliability, inter-rater reliability, content validity, and concurrent validity with the Life Satisfaction Index–Z are reported [107].

4. *The Role Activity Performance Scale* (RAPS) was developed by Good-Ellis, Fine, and Spencer as an evaluation of role performance for adult psychiatric patients [41]. A semistructured interview yields information in 12 areas (work or work equivalent, education, home management, nuclear and extended family relationships, mate relationship, parental role, social relationships, leisure activities, self-management, health-care role, hygiene and appearance, and rehabilitation treatment settings). Primary, secondary, and tertiary roles are identified for the 18-month period prior to treatment. Results are scored using an ordinal scale of 1 to 6, with 1 being the most functional. An overall score of role performance can be calculated. Administration and scoring protocols are provided. Preliminary studies suggest that some roles have concurrent validity with the Social Adjustment Scale–II, the Global Assessment Scale (GAS), and DSM III, Axis 5 [41].

5. *The Adolescent Role Assessment* (ARA) was developed by Black as an evaluation of inpatient adolescents' past and present role performance and the resulting effects on occupational choice [15]. It yields information on childhood play, socialization with family, peers, and at school, as well as occupational choice and work. Behaviors are judged appropriate, marginal, or inappropriate. Administration protocol and guidelines for rating behavior are provided.

6. *The Routine Task History* (RTH) was developed by Allen as an initial interview for acutely ill adult psychiatric patients [2]. Based on the cognitive disabilities frame of reference, it yields information about the patient's living situation, social support, self-care responsibilities, work history, educational history, interests, recent typical day, past hospitalizations, and the patient's assessment of his assets, limitations, and goals. The administration protocol allows for tailoring questions to meet specific patient needs.

from reactivity: The process of recording a problem tends to change it in the desired direction [16]. For example, if you started recording every cigarette you smoked right when you smoked it, you would probably smoke fewer cigarettes. This tendency for reactivity makes self-monitoring an effective treatment strategy [8], but must be considered when using it for evaluation. Although self-monitoring has been reported as a viable evaluation instrument in many psychologic studies (see Barlow, Hayes, and Nelson's review [8, p. 97]), at this writing the use of self-monitoring as an evaluation instrument has not been reported in the psychiatric O.T. literature. Useful strategies for designing these instruments and increasing patient compliance should be reviewed before using them. Examples of self-monitoring instruments appear in Fig. 2-4.

Self-Report Instruments
Whereas self-monitoring requires the observation and recording of ongoing behavior, self-report instruments ask patients to remember and record their behaviors, feelings, and perceptions after the fact [16]. Self-reports are often criticized because their results may not always coincide with direct observations of the patient's behavior by another source. Nevertheless, self-reports are not inferior evaluation in-

Fig. 2-4. Examples of self-monitoring instruments.

Self-monitoring instruments are individually designed for each patient's specific problems. They are an organized record, kept by the patient, of events he considers relevant to his problem [16]. Self-monitoring instruments are of several types: frequency counts, self-ratings, and diaries or logs [8].

1. *Frequency counts.* Noting the number of times the behavior occurs is especially useful when the behavior is clear cut and well defined, such as obsessive thoughts, bulimic episodes, cigarettes smoked, or food eaten. An example of a frequency count follows [8]:

Time interval	Saturday	Sunday	Monday	Tuesday	Wednesday	Thursday	Friday
Midnight–6:00 AM							
6:00–8:00 AM							
8:00–10:00 AM							
10:00–noon							
Noon–2:00 PM							
2:00–4:00 PM							
4:00–6:00 PM							
6:00–8:00 PM							
8:00–10:00 PM							
10:00–midnight							
Daily Total							

Fig. 2-4 (continued)

2. *Self-ratings.* The qualitative aspects of a problem (such as intensity, amount, duration, or degree of distress) can be measured with a self-rating instrument. The more specific the problem, the more useful the instrument can be. Since self-ratings are generally brief and completed at the time the problem or behavior occurs, they have the potential for measuring the outcome of O.T. treatment.
Examples of self-rating scales follow:

Extent to which I feel I can be honest in group

1	2	3	4	5	6	7	8	9
Can never be honest			Can sometimes be honest					Can always be be completely honest

---

Feelings of depression

1	2	3	4	5	6	7	8	9
Not depressed		Slightly depressed		Moderately depressed		Strongly depressed		Severely depressed

---

3. *Diaries or patient logs.* Diaries allow the patient to identify the circumstances surrounding the occurrence of the problem in his everyday life. Monitored criteria include time of day, event, who was there, what patient said (or felt), events that followed, and patient's reaction to the event. Rating scales are often combined with the log to have the patient rate his feelings about the incident. Examples of diaries follow:

Patient's name _____ Day and date _____

Time	Incident	Depression scale rating	Your reaction
_____	_____	_____	_____
_____	_____	_____	_____
_____	_____	_____	_____
_____	_____	_____	_____
_____	_____	_____	_____

Assertiveness Situations
Date and time:

Situation:

What did you do?

What were you thinking?

How did the situation end?

How did you feel about the outcome?
  (0 = very dissatisfied; 10 = very satisfied)

---

struments; they simply measure different variables. "Self-report assesses what the patient says about what he or she is thinking, feeling, or doing" [8, p. 145], and this may not always match how he appears to an external observer. Self-report is particularly useful to evaluate the patient's subjective experiences and thoughts, such as negative self-statements or obsessions. Actual motor behavior can be observed by others; yet self-report instruments can provide the patient's views about this behavior.

Self-report instruments are fairly easy to use and often can be completed by the patient before he attends O.T., thus allowing the time in therapy to be used more efficiently. There are dozens of self-report instruments, but most can be classified as one of three types: questionnaires, checklists, and anchored rating scales.

1. *Questionnaires.* Questionnaires usually list a variety of questions that require short answers. They are probably the most frequently used self-report instrument [8]. Like interviews, they have many applications for a variety of problems and are applicable to most frames of reference. For example, the Activity Configuration [28] and The Self-Directed Search [50] are questionnaires frequently used in psychiatric O.T.
2. *Checklists.* Various items, such as problems, situations, thoughts, feelings, or values, are listed on a checklist; the patient is asked to indicate those that apply to him. The length of the response required from the patient is short: either it applies or it does not. Checklists do not usually measure the intensity, frequency, or duration of the item, just whether or not it eixsts for that patient. Checklists used in O.T. include the Interest Checklist [73] and the Role Checklist [11].
3. *Anchored rating scales.* Unlike checklists, anchored rating scales measure the qualitative aspects of the problem, such as intensity, frequency, or duration. Anchored scales are designed with a range of possible responses in equal increments between the two end points [16]. One end point represents the high side of the scale, and other other represents the low side of the scale. Patients mark the response that most closely matches their perceptions. The inclusion of five to nine points on the scale is recommended; any more or less makes it difficult to discriminate accurately. Anchored rating scales used in O.T. include the Leisure Satisfaction Index [13] and the Life Attitude Profile [91].

As with interviews and self-monitoring instruments, self-reports have several limitations. The patient must be able to cooperate and provide reliable information, and self-report instruments are especially prone to response bias and social desirability [16]. Response bias refers to the tendency to answer items in a patterned manner, such as marking every item false or giving every item the same numeric rating. Social desirability refers to the tendency to answer items with the perceived socially acceptable response. For instance, "Is your dad a hard worker?" implies a socially acceptable answer. The patient may choose the expected answer even though it may not reflect his actual perception. These limitations can be reduced, in part, by careful phrasing and sequencing of the items on the instrument. The most effective way to minimize these limitations involves the manner in which you present the instrument to the patient. "The way you involve someone in completing a measure is probably as important as selecting just the right measure for them to fill out" [16, p. 143]. Bloom and Fischer suggest several strategies you can use to increase the accuracy of your data from self-report instruments [16].

1. *Explain the purpose.* Take time to go over the purpose of the instrument; what it means, how it will be used, and why you need the information. Assure the person that the information you are collecting will be actually used in planning his

treatment. Remind him that truthful, accurate information on his part is needed for you to be best able to help him.

2. *Explain the procedure.* Make sure the patient understands what he is expected to do. Does he understand how to fill out the instrument? Are there any items he does not understand? Is he aware of when it is supposed to be finished? Does he have all the materials he needs, such as pencils and notebooks, on hand?

3. *Anticipate difficulties.* Be as sensitive as possible to your patient's educational, social, and cultural background. Some persons may be uncomfortable with self-report instruments. Failure to address this issue with the patient may lead to incomplete or distorted answers. Limited reading comprehension and visual impairment also affect accuracy. Be prepared to read the questionnaire to your patient and record his answers, if necessary.

Self-report instruments are useful to evaluate your patient's subjective and cognitive perceptions [8,16]. They are not adequate as a single source of evaluation data. Used in conjunction with other evaluations, however, they provide valuable input about your patient's perspective on his problems. Selected self-report instruments are described in Figure 2-5.

Fig. 2-5. Examples of self-report instruments.

Questionnaires

1. *The Activity Configuration* has been in clinical use for many years in various forms. Cynkin refined a questionnaire (interview, if given orally) for use with various patient populations [28]. It yields information on values, educational and work history, and vocational interests and plans. Variations include use of activities clock (or pie of life). At this writing, no standardization data have been established on any of these instruments.

2. *The Self-directed Search* (SDS) was developed by Holland as a self-administered, self-scored, and self-interpreted exploration of vocational possibilities [50]. Instrument yields information about the match between the person's activities, competencies, and self-estimates and various occupational groups. SDS uses typology of person, environments, and interactions to suggest how to make vocational choices. Six personality types are identified: realistic (frank, persistent, practical, modest); investigative (analytic, cautious, intellectual, rational, independent); artistic (complicated, emotional, expressive, idealistic, intuitive); social (cooperative, convincing, helpful, insightful, kind); enterprising (adventurous, energetic, optimistic, self-confident); and conventional (conforming, conscientious, orderly, calm, efficient). Results are summarized in a three-letter code identifying congruent personality types. The code is used to locate suitable occupations in an accompanying booklet, *The Occupations Finder*. Administration and scoring protocols are provided. Instrument has been tested extensively and used in hundreds of studies. Norms are provided, and all forms of reliability and validity are established. Instrument has particularly strong construct and predictive validity [50].

Checklists

1. *The Interest Checklist* (IC) has been in clinical use for many years in many forms. Matsutsuyu developed a checklist for psychiatric inpatients that is useful with all frames of reference [73]. It yields information on number and type of activities as well as degree of interest. Rogers, Weinstein, and Figone refined the checklist, added a 5-point scale to indicate degree of interest, and sorted interests into five categories with operational definitions: activities of daily living (basic domestic arts), manual skills (activities using hands to make a finished product), cultural/educational (training, development, and refinement of mind through systematic study), physical sports (games/play requiring physical strength or stamina), and social recreation (activities involving others pursued for pleasure). Test-retest reliability was high with high school seniors. Initial study suggests some construct validity of the cultural/educational and physical sports categories with adolescents [94].

Fig. 2-5 (continued)

2. *The Role Checklist* (RC) was developed by Oakley as an evaluation of role participation for adolescent, adult, and elderly patients with various problems [11]. Based on the model of human occupation, it yields information on the patient's perception of his participation in various roles throughout his life, his role balance and continuity, and the degree to which each role is valued over time. Information is gathered on 11 roles (student, worker, volunteer, caregiver, home maintainer, friend, family member, religious participant, hobbyist/amateur, participant in organizations, and other). Instrument is divided into two parts: participation in roles (past, present, future) and degree of value of roles (not important, somewhat important, very important). An administration protocol is provided. Preliminary data suggest test-retest reliability, face and content validity, and ability to discriminate between patients with adaptive and maladaptive role behaviors [11].

Anchored Scales
1. *The Leisure Satisfaction Index* (LSI) was developed by Beard and Ragheb to evaluate the extent to which people perceive certain needs as satisfied through leisure activities [13]. It addresses psychologic, educational, social, relaxational, physiologic, and aesthetic needs. An administration protocol is provided. Face and content validity are reported [13].
2. *The Life Attitude Profile* (LAP) was developed by Reker and Peacock as a multidimensional instrument to measure attitudes toward life [91]. Based on Frankl's Logotherapy [39], this instrument yields information in three major areas: degree of existential meaning and purpose in life, strength of motivation to find meaning, and acceptance in the present of future potential. Seven subscales are identified: life purpose (zest for life, contentment with life, excitement, fulfillment, and meaningfulness); existential vacuum (lack of meaning and purpose in life, lack of goals, tension, frustration, meaningless, free-floating anxiety); life control (personal responsibility, freedom to make life choices, perception of internal control of life events); death acceptance (lack of fear and an anxiety about death and dying); will to meaning (transcendent consciousness, stirring to find concrete meaning in personal existence, appreciation of life beyond immediate given, search for ideals and values); goal seeking (desire to achieve new goals in the future, to search for new and different experiences, to be on the move); and meaning to fulfill (future fulfillment, acceptance of future potential, positive expectations of oneself and one's life, hopefulness, personal optimism). Administration and scoring protocols and preliminary norms (mean, but no standard deviation) are provided. Reasonable claims exist for test-retest reliability and face and content validity. Concurrent validity has been established with five scales: Dean's Alienation Scale, Reid-Ware Internal External Locus of Control, Lodzinski's Academic Goals Inventory, Time Competency subtest of Shostrom's Personal Orientation Inventory, and Crowne-Marlow Social Desirability Scale. Some preliminary evidence suggests that several subscales (goal seeking, life purpose, meaning to fulfill, and acceptance of death) can differentiate people at different developmental stages [91].

Behavior Ratings
Behavior ratings refer to structured observations of the patient by an observer who then rates the behavior on given criteria. Observations can be of several types: naturalistic, analogue, or participant monitoring [44,98].

1. *Naturalistic observation.* These observations take place in the patient's natural environment. They have been used successfully in a variety of settings and with different problems. Naturalistic observations are particularly useful in evaluating the outcome of treatment [44]. Observation of the patient at home determines if the skills learned in therapy have generalized to his life outside the treatment setting. Of all types of observation, it is the least subject to assumptions about the patient's ability to function at home because that is where he is observed. As you might guess, naturalistic observation is time-consuming and expensive; however, it is particularly useful for therapists working in home-health and community-based settings. What could be a better way to evaluate

kitchen safety, for instance, than to observe the person functioning in his own kitchen?

2. *Analogue observations.* These are observations of the patient's performance in a "created" environment by an objective observer [44]. For our purposes, analogue observations involve the observation and rating of the patient's performance in the O.T. clinic by a therapist (or student) other than the one who is treating him. Specific tasks to be used are not identified; any task normally used in the course of O.T. treatment is acceptable. Setting up the created environment—or in this case the task for the patient to perform in the O.T. clinic—increases the probability that a particular patient characteristic can be elicited and, therefore, observed and rated. Analogue observation rating scales in O.T. generally include ratings of the patient's general, task, and interpersonal behaviors. Examples of O.T. analogue observations and rating scales are the Comprehensive Occupational Therapy Evaluation (COTE) [21] and the Prevocational Assessment of Rehabilitation Potential (PARP) [30]. Analogue observations are more cost-effective than naturalistic observations. Nevertheless, because evaluating a patient in a created environment entails many confounding variables, the information gathered in analogue oservations can only be used to describe the patient's performance in that particular situation. The results do not generalize to global statements about the patient's overall performance. Analogue observations are most useful for ratings of here and now behavior, not global predictions of performance.

3. *Participant monitoring.* Participant monitoring involves observing the patient while you are actively working with him [98]. You might be assisting him with an activity, giving directions, or facilitating a group project while you are observing what he is saying and doing. This level of observation skill takes some practice to develop, as it requires concentration on two tasks simultaneously. Participant monitoring needs no special equipment or preparation; it can be done any time the patient is treated. Because it is fairly unobtrusive, the patient is often unaware that he is being observed, thus minimizing reactivity as a variable. Nevertheless, participant monitoring is very susceptible to observer bias [44]. Haynes suggests that the therapist's past interactions with the patient, preconceived ideas about the patient, and beliefs about the usefulness of the data being collected contribute to observer bias [44]. Rating-scale items that are vague and lack specific measurable qualities also incrase the chances of observer bias. For instance, "patient appears disheveled and unkempt" leaves much more room for personal interpretation than does "clothes clean, wrinkled, buttons missing, clothes not tucked in or zipped."

Behavior ratings are structured observations and ratings of your patient's performance. They can be most useful as indicators of the patient's present functioning in that test situation, rather than predictions of the patient's global performance. Selected behavior rating scales are described in Fig. 2-6.

Task Evaluations

Task evaluations also use created environments to elicit certain patient performances, but, unlike analogue observations, task evaluations specify the tasks to be used. Patient performances that might not otherwise occur or that may not occur with sufficient frequency to be assessed in the O.T. clinic are prompted and elicited by specific tasks. For example, the Bay Area Functional Performance Evaluation (BaFPE) [17] uses five tasks (sorting shells, money and marketing, home drawing, block design, and draw-a-person) to evaluate patient performance on 12 functional parameters (paraphrasing, decision making, motivation, organization of time and

Fig. 2-6. Examples of rating scales.

1. *The Comprehensive Occupational Therapy Evaluation* (COTE) was developed by Brayman, Kirby, Misenheimer, and Short as an initial evaluation and progress report of inpatients observed in O.T. [21]. Instrument yields information on three categories of behavior: general, interpersonal, and task. No administration protocol is suggested; any O.T. activity can be used with the instrument. Results are scored on a 5-point scale with 0 as normal. A scoring protocol is provided. Initial study suggests inter-rater reliability and that the COTE scores reflect changes in the patient's condition (that is, the scores are lower on discharge than on admission) [22].

2. *The Prevocational Assessment of Rehabilitation Potential* (PARP) was developed by Ethridge to evaluate the vocational potential of institutionalized psychiatric patients [30]. The patient's behavior is observed in routine O.T. groups and rated in four areas: work (motivation, initiative, ability to follow through, ability to take directions, quality of workmanship, quantity of work, attendance); socialization (participation in social activities, quantity and content of verbalization, aggressiveness, hostility, thoughtfulness, peer adjustment, ability to work with others); personality characteristics (unusual behavior, anxiety, judgment, frustration tolerance); and general observations (appearance, learning capacity, knowledge of equipment and safety, use of time). No administration protocol is supplied. The scoring protocol uses a 4-point scale with 4 as excellent. Initial study indicated that the PARP had some ability to predict which patients would be successfully rehabilitated (defined as one month of employment after discharge and "adequate adjustment to the community") [30].

Fig. 2-7. Examples of task evaluations.

1. *The Bay Area Functional Performance Evaluation* (BaFPE) was developed by Bloomer and Williams to evaluate the functional performance of adult psychiatric inpatients [17]. The instrument yields information on two scales: Task-Oriented Assessment (TOA) and the Social Interaction Scale (SIS). The TOA uses five tasks (sorting shells, money and marketing, home drawing, block design, and draw-a-person) to evaluate 10 functional parameters (paraphrasing, decision making, motivation, organization of time and material, mastery and self-esteem, frustration tolerance, attention span, ability to abstract, verbal or behavioral evidence of thought or mood disorder, and ability to follow instructions leading to correct task completion). SIS uses a rating scale to measure seven functional parameters (response to authority figures, verbal communication, psychomotor behavior, independence/dependence, socially appropriate behavior, ability to work with peers, and participation in group or program activities). Administration and scoring protocols are supplied. Initial normative data on both patient and normal populations are given. Inter-rater reliability as well as face and content validity are reported [18]. Preliminary study suggests construct validity and concurrent validity with the GAS and the Functional Life Scale. Changes in patient's condition were reflected by the BaFPE (that is, scores were higher on discharge than on admission). Revisions made in the BaFPE are currently under study. Standardization data were collected on initial research edition. Revisions of the TOA include the addition of two functional parameters (time needed to complete and cognitive functioning). The language has been simplified and the tasks clarified and refined. Changes have been made on the scoring forms to make the instrument easier to use. Revisions of the SIS include (a) the addition of multiple situational observations for rating (one-to-one interactions, mealtimes, unstructured groups in common living areas, activity groups, verbal groups), (b) making two parameters bidirectional (independence/dependence and hyper-/hypoactive behavior), and (c) obtaining a self-report of social skills [19].

2. *The Scorable Self-Care Evaluation* (SCCE) was developed by Clark and Peters to evaluate work, daily living, and leisure self-care activities in adults with various problems [25]. It yields quantifiable scores on four self-care scales: personal care (initial appearance, orientation, hygiene, communication, first aid); housekeeping (food selection, household chores, safety, laundry); work and leisure (leisure activity, transportation, job-seeking skills); and financial management (making change, keeping a checking account, paying personal bills, budgeting, procurement of supplemental income, source of income). Results are scored with points given for errors; total score

is calculated. Administration and scoring protocols are supplied. Initial normative data were established with a normal population. Preliminary data suggest test-retest reliability on three of the four scales (personal care was the exception). Inter-rater reliability was adequate. There are some claims to face and content validity.

3. *The Kohlman Evaluation of Living Skills* (KELS) was designed by McGourty (née Kohlman) to evaluate rapidly basic living skills in acutely ill adult psychiatric patients [75]; it can also be used with other populations. Instrument yields information about functional performance in five areas: self-care (appearance, frequency of self-care activities), safety and health (dangerous household situations, first-aid actions, knowledge of emergency numbers, knowledge of medical and dental facilities), money management (making change, source of income, food stamps, food budgeting, budgeting of monthly income, banking, paying bills), transportation and telephone (mobility in community, use of public transportation, use of telephone book), work and leisure (plans for future employment, leisure activity involvement). Administration and scoring protocols are supplied. Preliminary normative data were collected on acutely ill psychiatric inpatients. The instrument is currently under revision.

4. *The Allen Cognitive Level* (ACL) was developed by Allen and refined by Moore as an initial evaluation of the cognitive level of acutely ill adult psychiatric patients [2]. The instrument identifies the degree of complexity of a leather lacing stitch that the patient is able to imitate. Results are rated on a scale of 1 to 6 with 6 as the highest cognitive functioning. Each rating has an accompanying description of task behavior in three major areas: attention, motor actions, and conscious awareness. Administration and scoring protocols are provided. Initial studies suggest inter-rater reliability, predictive validity in placing patients in O.T. groups, and concurrent validity with brief psychiatric rating scale. Improvement in patient's condition was reflected in ACL scores (that is, scores were higher at discharge than on admission) [2].

materials, mastery and self-esteem, frustration tolerance, attention span, ability to abstract, verbal or behavioral evidence of thought or mood disorder, ability to follow instructions leading to correct task completion, time needed to complete, and cognitive functioning [19]. Because the performance of these five tasks is believed to require the 12 stated behaviors (functional parameters), the patient's actual use of these behaviors can be observed and rated. Task evaluations are convenient, more economical than naturalistic observations, and useful in providing information about the patient's actual ability to perform. Nevertheless, information gathered from task evaluations must be interpreted with care. Content and criterion validity are especially important to establish for task evaluations. Without them, you cannot be sure whether the tasks used on the evaluation really elicited and adequately measured the behaviors you thought they were measuring. Unless predictive validity has been established, task evaluations are most accurately interpreted as an indication of the patient's performance in that setting at that time. Predicting whether the patient's performance will generalize to other settings based on the results of the task evaluation alone is not advised.

In summary, task evaluations measure identified patient performances (functional parameters) that can be elicited by specific tasks. Unlike behavior-rating scales, task evaluations specify the task to be used. They are one of our major evaluation tools; however, they need to be interpreted with caution. Selected task evaluations are described in Fig. 2-7.

Neuropsychologic Instruments
Growing interest in the sensory integration frame of reference has spawned several evaluations of neuropsychologic functioning of persons with psychiatric disorders. These evaluations, such as the SBC [96], include both physical measurements of function (such as strength, range of motion, and hand grip) and performance of tasks requiring several skills (such as Kephart's circles and drawing persons). Al-

Fig. 2-8. Examples of
neuropsychological
instruments.

1. *The SBC Adult Psychiatric Sensory Integration Evaluation* was developed by Schroeder, Block, Trottier (née Campbell), and Stowell to evaluate comprehensively adult psychiatric patients' sensorimotor functioning [97]. The instrument yields information in three major areas: sensorimotor responses (eye-hand-foot dominance, posture, neck rotation, gait, hand observation, grip strength, fine motor control, diadochokinesis, finger-thumb opposition, visual pursuits, upper extremity (UE) bilateral coordination, crossing midline, UE stability, trunk stability, classic Romberg, sharpened Romberg, overflow movements, neck righting, rolling, asymmetric tonic neck reflex, symmetric tonic reflex, tonic labyrinthine reflex, protective extension, seated equilibrium, body image), abnormal movements resulting from illness or medication, and self-reported childhood history (general history, delayed development, neurologic soft signs, and hyperactivity) [96]. Results are scored on a 4-point scale, with 0 representing no difficulty with task. Administration and scoring protocols are supplied. Initial studies indicate inter-rater reliability except in the areas of abnormal movements and rolling [97].

2. *The Person Symbol* (PS) in the form of draw-a-person has been used clinically for years by different professions. It has been used as a measure of mental maturity, as a projective test (frequently by psychologists as part of the house-tree-person instrument), and as a diagnostic tool. King refined the PS for use with adult psychiatric patients as an evaluation of neurologic and psychologic organization [64]. The instrument yields information on body concept (cognitive aspects, as a reflection of own physical status); sensory-integrative dysfunction (equilibrium responses, shoulder girdle stability, midline problems, tactile responsiveness); organicity; and sexual identity. Results are rated using the Goodenough-Harris Rating Scale (GHRS), and include the number of incorporated details, appropriateness of proportions, and accurate depiction of joints and movement. The GHRS has acceptable inter-rater reliability and concurrent validity with other measures of mental ability. Norms are provided for children; however, preliminary studies by King indicate that the GHRS will accommodate adult performance [64]. Administration protocol is provided. Initial studies of PS and GHRS with psychiatric patients suggest satisfactory inter-rater reliability and concurrent validity with the NOSIE-30. Beginning normative data were collected on both patient and normal populations. Data suggest that PS reflects changes in the patient's condition (improved body concept with clinical improvement) [64].

though these evaluations directly measure the patient's neuropsychologic functioning, they are also constrained by the same limitations as task evaluations. Selected neuropsychologic evaluations are described in Fig. 2-8.

Projective Instruments

Projective instruments are a form of task evaluation that uses media, usually unstructured, to evaluate the patient's task behaviors (e.g., attention, problem solving, frustration tolerance) and psychologic functioning (e.g., personality characteristics, needs, unconscious conflicts, and symbol production) [48]. Projective instruments require that the patient generate material on his own with a minimum of structure or direction from the therapist. Their function is similar to that of open-indirect questions in an interview. Although they can provide information that you may not have thought to ask for, they are lengthy and produce so much information that they are often unwieldy and difficult to synthesize.

Projective instruments are part of our psychiatric O.T. heritage. They do, however, entail a number of serious limitations and precautions. Except for the B. H. Battery, the functional components measured by projective instruments are generally not specifically defined [46]. Observations and ratings of a patient's performance are thus based on the therapist's judgment. In addition, projective assessments often use symbol production as a measure of intrapsychic conflict. Although endorsed by the psychodynamic frame of reference, therapist interpretation of the patient's symbols is risky. Without extensive training in symbol analysis, it is questionable whose symbols are being interpreted—the patient's or the therapist's. The story is told of a psychiatric resident who came into the O.T. clinic to observe. Noticing the paintings drying on the wall, he asked who had done the one painted all in black. When told the patient's name, the resident exclaimed, "Look at all the repressed anger and hostility in that picture!" He noted that he had worked for months with that patient to get in touch with those feelings, and he proclaimed the occupational therapist a miracle worker in facilitating the breakthrough. Grateful that the value of O.T. was finally being recognized, yet nagged by her conscience, the therapist finally told the resident that perhaps the patient did indeed have repressed anger and hostility, but his choice of black paint was due to his inability to reach any other color from where he was sitting at the table! As Sigmund Freud reportedly said when asked to expound on the symbolic significance of his ever-present cigar, "Sometimes a cigar is just a cigar." Because of their length, projective instruments have limited usefulness in acute treatment facilities. Finally, since the purpose of the evaluation is not readily obvious to the patient and may seem unrelated to his immediate problems, projective evaluations are frequently refused. With few exceptions, most of the patient performances addressed by projective instruments can be evaluated in other ways that are more direct, accurate, and cost-effective. Whether or not they should remain an important facet of O.T. in psychiatry is an issue ripe for scholarly debate. Selected projective instruments are described in Fig. 2-9.

Selecting an Instrument(s)

How do you select an instrument? Just as you would not use a hammer to crack an egg, you should not use an instrument outside its stated purpose. Instruments are usually not generic; they do not fit all patients, with all problems, in all types of settings. If misused, they can provide inaccurate and misleading data. Selecting appropriate instrument(s) requires several steps (see Fig. 2-10).

Fig. 2-9. Examples of projective instruments.

1. *The Collage* has been used in clinical practice in various forms for many years. Buck and Provancher used the collage as an evaluation tool [24]; Lerner et al. refined it to evaluate psychologic processes in acutely ill psychiatric inpatients [66]. An administration protocol is supplied [24, 66]; and a scoring protocol has been developed [67]. Collages are scored in three areas: formal variables (color of paper, number of pictures, color of most cuttings, overall color effect, manner in which cuttings are made, degree of neatness, pictures upside down or sideways, overlapping pictures, pictures glued completely over others, overall balance, fragmentation, dimensionalization, cutting out words, framing), content variables (number, age, and sex of persons; feelings expressed; activities shown; emphasis on body parts; unusual dress; central theme; number of animals; emphasis on objects; types of objects; appropriate title), and patient-therapist variables (seeks repetition of directions, seeks reassurance, time taken to complete). Initial studies suggest inter-rater reliability and face and content validity when collage is used to make descriptive and dynamic inferences by experienced psychiatric staff [67]. One study reported corresponding change of collage score with degree of clinical improvement [66]. Preliminary study of construct validity suggests that some variables on collage distinguish between psychiatric patients and "normal" people [67].
2. *The B. H. Battery* was developed by Hemphill to evaluate task skills and level of psychologic functioning and to assist in the diagnosis of, and treatment planning for, psychiatric inpatients. It is recommended that the battery be given 24 hours after admission [47]. Two tasks are used (mosaic tiling and fingerpainting) to evaluate seven task and psychologic behaviors (use of color, approach to the medium, use of space, form, strokes, characteristic of the design, verbalization during the activity, and theme). Administration and scoring protocols are provided [46]. Initial study suggests inter-rater reliability [47].

Fig. 2-10. A guide for selecting the appropriate instrument.

Use the following questions as a guide to select the instrument(s) you will use to evaluate your patient's performance further.

1. What specific problem areas require further evaluation?

2. Which of the instrument categories would best measure this area of function for your patient?

3. What is the basis for that opinion?

4. Of the instrument categories you identified, which specific instruments are recommended by the frame of reference you are using with this patient? (Frame of reference: _____)

5. What are the practical constraints of your treatment facility that have an impact on the instrument(s) you select?

6. Which instrument(s) will you use to evaluate your patient further?

7. What is the basis for that selection?

Define Patient Problem Areas

What are the patient's specific areas of functioning that need further evaluation? Based on the data base you collected in the screening process, identify those areas that you suspect are problematic, but about which you do not have enough information to define the problem in detail. Review all the areas of functioning included in the domain of concern as interpreted by the frame of reference you selected. Which of these are problematic for your patient?

Identify Instrument Categories

Before trying to pick out specific instrument(s) to use, identify which categories of instruments (discussed in this section) are best suited to measure each particular problem area. For instance, if you wanted to evaluate your patient's ability to handle his own banking, you would select interview, self-report, or task as appropriate categories of instruments. You thus could ask the person about his abilities, have him fill out a questionnaire, or actually fill out a check and deposit slip. At this point, the patient's needs determine the type(s) of instruments you would use. If the patient were able to provide a reliable self-report, the interview and questionnaire might be sufficient. However, questions about the reliability of the patient's self-report would indicate the use of an interview and task evaluation.

Select Specific Instruments

Finally, you select the specific instrument(s) you will use to evaluate your patient. This decision is based on several factors:

1. *Frame of reference.* It does not make sense to use one frame of reference for the screening and then switch to another when selecting evaluations. As you recall, one of the purposes of a frame of reference is to provide guidance and structure to assessment and treatment planning. Once you pick a frame of reference, stick with it throughout the whole process. Although instruments from other frames of reference might provide interesting information, most of it is unusable to you because it falls outside the concepts of the frame of reference you chose to use. Picking and choosing among frames of reference at this point in the process is similar to not using one at all.

2. *Practical constraints.* The practical constraints of the treatment facility influence the instruments you select. For instance, if the time you have to evaluate and treat the patient is limited, you would select the briefest and the minimal number of evaluations required so you would have time for treatment. Similarly, the size of your case load and the availability of space and equipment also influence your selection of an instrument.

3. *Other factors.* Given the choice of several instruments, select the one(s) with the most standardization data. (Standardization data for the O.T. instruments described are summarized in Table 2-1, p. 70.) As you learned in the section on "Principles of Measurement" (p. 64), instrument development is a lengthy and complex process [14]. Although self-developed instruments seem to be common [58], nonstandardized instruments carry severe limitations that impair their usefulness. The more standardization information you have about an instrument, the more confidence you can place in your results. Finally, how many instruments should you use? Attempt to limit it to the minimum needed to collect enough information for effective treatment planning. As you proceed with treatment, other areas may be identified for evaluation. Is one evaluation enough? Certainly using more than one instrument to measure a problem increases your accuracy [29,65,82,109], yet using multiple instruments also increases the chances of interactional effects between instruments that can confound your results (type I error) [106]. This issue is discussed further in the section on "Sources of Error" (p. 96). Effective evaluation of patient performance, then, involves a balance between gathering just enough data to plan treatment, but not so much that you alienate your patient, gather irrelevant information, or suffer from data overload (a condition marked by inability to make sense of all the information you have).

Instrument development in psychiatric O.T. is proceeding at an encouraging pace. Although it is tempting to try the latest evaluation the minute it comes in the mail, get in the habit of reading and reviewing the instrument critically so you can use it most effectively. Try it out several times on your colleagues, friends, and family to make sure you are familiar with the protocol before you begin. Evaluation instruments add critically important information to your data base, but only when they are selected and used appropriately.

Your Turn

It is time for a review of your newly acquired knowledge. For each instrument category, write a brief description including its purpose, strengths, and limitations. List one specific O.T. instrument for each category. Although all of this information has been given, thinking it through and writing it for yourself will help you to integrate it.

Interviews:

Example of interview:

Self-monitoring instruments:

Example of self-monitoring instrument:

Self-report instruments:

Example of self-report instrument:

Behavior rating:

Example of behavior rating:

Task evaluation:

Example of task evaluation:

Neuropsychologic instruments:

Example of neuropsychologic instrument:

Projective instruments:

Example of projective instrument:

Summary
This section looked at evaluation as a two-step process. The first step is understanding the principles of measurement, or what an instrument is designed to do, what you can expect of it, and how much confidence you can place in its results. The second is making an informed selection based on familiarity with the evaluation instruments available. Discriminating selection, appropriate use, and substantiated interpretation of instruments represent sound evaluation practices. Once you have all the data, you need to synthesize it and identify the problems you will treat in O.T.

Data Synthesis and Interpretation

Synthesizing and interpreting the data you have collected so far to determine your patient's problems and strengths completes the assessment process. Rogers suggests that at this point a shift in your thinking occurs from the classic, textbook picture of the disorder to the disorder as experienced and exhibited by your patient [92]. The frame of reference you selected delineates criteria for determining both functional and dysfunctional behavior. Application of these criteria to the data base you have collected helps you identify your patient's specific problems and strengths.

Identifying Problems

Several factors influence your identification of problems. Problems are a behavior, thought, feeling, activity, or situation that is of concern to both you and the patient [16]. Problems do not always indicate the absolute lack of something; sometimes they involves a strength that needs further development. For instance, your patient may assertively initiate contacts with persons of the opposite sex sometimes, but not frequently or consistently enough to be satisfactory to him. The problem, then, is to increase the strength of this assertive behavior to a satisfactory level. Additionally, not all dysfunctional behaviors that you identify as problems are perceived by the patient as problematic. So, although you may have identified an inconsistency in your patient's use of his leisure time, he may not see that as a problem. Finally, not all the patient's problems (sexual performance dysfunction, for instance) are appropriate for O.T. treatment. Identifying problems, then, involves synthesizing the raw data into a list of problems and strengths, discussing the problems with your patient, and deciding which problems are appropriate to address in O.T. (see Tables 2-2 to 2-5 for examples).

The first step is to synthesize the data. The following section draws heavily on the work of Bloom and Fischer in evaluating outcome of therapy [16]. They suggest that problem identification requires two processes: specificity and prioritization of the list of problems.

Table 2-2. Examples of problems, indicators, and strengths: Functional performance

Area of function	Problem	Indicators	Strengths
Social	Not assertive in making friends	No contacts initiated in past month (self-report)	Having friends is valued
		Low score on assertiveness scale (self-report)	
		High degree of discomfort when speaking to people (self-monitoring and behavior rating)	
Cognitive	Difficulty making decisions	Unable to choose between two tasks or two colors (task)	Has job
			Has functioned well in past
		Written notice of work performance decline from supervisor (interview)	Increased functioning is valued

Table 2-2 (continued)

Area of function	Problem	Indicators	Strengths
Motor	Limited endurance	Four hours out of bed and involved in activity daily (self-monitoring Level of perceived fatigue after activities (self-monitoring, rating)	Muscle strength and Range of Motion (ROM) are adequate
Psychological	Feels inferior to peers	Has not initiated contact with peers in past 6 months (self-report, interview) High number of negative self-statements (self-monitoring) No activities done with peers in the past 6 months (self-report)	Having friends is valued Continues to attend school Has interests that can provide contact with peers
Sensory integration	Poor balance in physical activities	Loses balance when doing large motor activities (rating and self-report) Stumbles and loses balance when trying to walk fast	Strength and endurance are adequate Sitting balance is adequate

Compiled from Clark [26], Clark [27], Fidler [33], Fidler and Fidler [36], and Mosey [79].

Area of function	Problem	Indicators	Strengths
Vestibular and proprioceptive	Impaired balance	Protective extension elicited 3/4 trials Lost balance on Romberg 4/4 trials Unable to hold the sharpened Romberg for 10 seconds (neuropsychologic)	Strength and sitting balance are adequate
Tactile	Tactile defensiveness	Negative response to light quick touch (rating, interview) Short attention span Easily distracted (rating)	Able to tolerate touch when self-administered
Tactile/vestibular proprioceptive	Impaired bilateral coordination	Unable to draw Kephart circles in 3/3 trials Does not cross midline Does not discriminate between right and left sides of body (neuropsychologic)	Muscle strength and fine motor coordination adequate

Table 2-3. Examples of problems, indicators, and strengths: Sensory integration

Compiled from Ayers [5a], Hinajosa, et al [49], King [61], King [64a], Mack, Lindquist, and Parham [71,72], Schroeder and Herbert [95a], and Schroeder et al [96].

Table 2-4. Examples of problems, indicators, and strengths: Model of human occupation

Area of function	Problem	Indicators	Strengths
Volition	Feels loss of control over life	Externally oriented (self-report) Low number of independent decisions made in child care in past month (self-report, interview)	Believes in own skills in some areas such as leisure interests
Habituation	Current role performance imbalance	Low-satisfaction with role performance (self-report, interview) Discrepancy between valued roles and actual current participation (self-report, interview)	Has variety of valued roles Has history of successful role performance
Skills	Decreased concentration	Dissatifaction with level of concentration when reading (self-monitoring) Grades have gone from B to C this semester (interview)	No difficulty with eyes (no blurry or double vision)
Environment	Little interaction with other people outside of family	Uses only two environments: work and home (self-report) Experiences high degree of anxiety when attending new places besides home and work (self-monitoring and rating)	Has interests Involvement with others is valued

Compiled from Barris, Kielhofner, and Watts [10], Kielhofner [57], Mack, Lindquist, and Parham [71,72], and Nelville [81A].

Table 2-5. Examples of problems, indicators, and strengths: Cognitive disabilities

Area of function	Problem	Indicators	Strengths
Attention	Awareness of objects limited to visual cues	Does not identify or look for objects when hidden or covered up Color and form are the only two visual cues used (rating and task)	Attention is captured by sample; wishes to imitate
Attention	Does not attend to abstract, related properties of objects	Does not notice or use abstract spatial relationships (e.g., overlapping equally or leaving spaces between objects) Abstract relationships are not understood when explained (rating and task)	Attention is directed to one cue at a time

continued

Area of function	Problem	Indicators	Strengths	Table 2-5 *(continued)*
Motor actions	Does not invent new motor actions	Does not correct errors even with demonstrated solutions	Actions are goal directed	
		Unable to retain two-step directions (rating and task)		
Conscious awareness	Attention span limited to the immediate goal	Unable to maintain interest in the activity beyond one or two sessions	Complies with demonstrated procedure to reach goal	
		Measures time by individual needs such as time for lunch or time for medication (rating and task)		

Source: Allen, C. K. [2].

Specificity

Being specific means to state your patient's problem in precise enough terms that it can be observed and measured. Vague statements such as "poor self-esteem" and "inadequate social skills" reflect your interpretation of data without indicating the actual basis for this opinion. This failure to state specifics prohibits effective treatment because you have no idea of who, how, when, where, and under what circumstances these problems occur. Vague problems denote vague treatment goals (to improve self-esteem or to improve social skills), vague treatment methods (esteem-building activities or social skills training), and vague measures of treatment outcome (seemed to improve).

Stating specific problems includes identifying two components: the general topic of concern and specific indicators. The general topic of concern identifies the problem (e.g., feels dissatisfied with school), and the specific indicator(s) address how, when, where, and under what circumstances the problem occurs for that patient (e.g., tardy at school 75 percent of the time, grade average has decreased from B to C−). Problem indicators are based on the information gathered in the assessment, such as results of interviews, instruments, or reports from significant others. Stating more than one indicator for each problem helps to increase your specificity and the accuracy of your problem definition, as it requires you to find more than one indication of the problem. Problems and their related indicator(s) are individualized and reflect each patient's unique circumstances and personality. Although the general area of concern may apply to many patients, the specific indicator(s) may differ with each patient. For example:

Patient A
Problem — Difficulty making decisions
Indicator — Has not made homemaking decisions (menu planning, food or clothes shopping) without help from spouse in past month
Self-reports that dressing each day takes an hour because of indecision about what to wear

Patient B
Problem — Difficulty making decisions
Indicators — Six absences from work in past month
Reports from supervisor of failure to meet work deadlines
Has not paid bills for past 2 months

Patient C

Problem	Difficulty making decisions
Indicators	Self-reported failure to make disciplinary decisions with children
	Has not made breakfast or sent children off to school in past month

As you can see, the general problem can be shared by several persons, but the indicators are specific to each patient. Indicators are not pulled out of thin air; they are derived from information in the data base you collected. Additionally, the frame of reference used in the treatment planning process provides a structure within which to interpret this information. What might be indicators of *difficulty making decisions* in one frame of reference could be indicators of *cognitive disabilities* or *role disabilities* in other frames of reference. In other words, definition of problems and their indicator(s) reflects your patient's needs as interpreted by the frame of reference you have selected to guide your treatment (see Tables 2-2 to 2-5). Problem statements with specific indicators are a declaration of "what is" in precise, measurable terms. The success of your treatment will largely depend on the specificity of the problems and indicators [29,65,82,109].

Writing specific problems and indicators requires vigilance in eliminating vague statements. Check the specificity of your problem statements and indicators by asking yourself the following questions.

IS THE PROBLEM CLEAR?

When discussing a problem with your patient, ask for a concrete example to increase its clarity. Helpful questions to ask are: When does it occur? What times are the most bothersome for you? How long does it happen? Clarity of the problem indicators can be increased by asking your patient to define acceptable evidence to indicate that the problem has been resolved. For example, if the problem were "feels fearful," with acceptable resolution of "shopping alone in the shopping mall for 45 minutes," then possible indicators of the problem could be "does not shop alone at malls," or "high number of self-reported fearful feelings when in public." Just one reminder: in the pursuit of clarity, do not forget the cautions against bombarding your patient with multiple questions. Take the time to respond to your patient's responses before asking another question.

CAN THE PROBLEM BE OBSERVED?

Observability, in this case, means that the problem can be measured. It does not automatically imply that the problem must be an overt performance. Many problems are internal thoughts and feelings that only your patient can observe. Yet even internal problems (covert performances) can be defined with specific enough indicators that the person observing knows exactly what to look for. For example, poor self-esteem is difficult to measure, but negative self-statements can be self-monitored for their types and frequency. Poor hygiene is a conclusion; however, frequency of bathing and washing hair and clothes can be readily observed. Covert performances can have three types of indicators: overt behaviors (things you can see), self-monitored responses (patient's perceptions of the problem), or scores on an instrument. Taken together, they are assumed adequately to indicate the presence of a covert performance.

IS THE PROBLEM REIFIED?

Reification refers to the tendency to treat abstract concepts as though they were real-life things [16]. For example, both of the following statements contain reifications: "Joe has difficulty with authority figures because he is aggressive," and "Mary is splitting the staff because she is a borderline." Both the behavior and the offered explanation are abstract concepts that are treated like real things. *Difficulty with authority figures, aggressiveness, splitting the staff,* and *borderline* do not describe specific behaviors that indicate how, when, where, and under what circumstances the problem occurs. They are thus reified abstractions. Reified problems are sneaky. They sound good, and you have a vague idea what they mean, but precision is lacking. Unfortunately, psychiatric jargon contains numerous reifications. Inexperienced therapists are frequently bedazzled by the jargon spoken at staffing meetings. As one therapist put it, "I recognized the words, but didn't understand what was said." It is tempting to succumb to jargon (after all, you want to show everyone you know how to speak it, too), but it has no place when identifying problems. Weeding out your reifications takes vigilance. Although reifications cannot be treated, you can treat the problems implied by the reifications. Reifications are corrected by turning each abstraction into an adjective. "Joe is aggressive" is therefore rephrased as "Joe is demonstrating aggressive behaviors." If you then specify indicators for these aggressive behaviors, you will have stamped out a reification.

A list of a few suggested problems, possible indicators, and strengths by frame of reference appear in Tables 2-2 through 2-5. These are not intended to be exhaustive lists. Use them only to supply ideas for wording and format when writing your list of problems. Categories of evaluation instruments that supplied data are listed in parentheses after the problem indicators.

Prioritization

Listing all the problems you could treat is overwhelming for both you and the patient. Lack of treatment priorities defuses your efforts and reduces your chances of a successful outcome. Trying to treat all of the patient's problems at once requires that you either give minimal attention to each problem (most likely making little headway) or you sign up the patient for a lengthy course of treatment. Noting the tendency of occupational therapists to do the latter, a perceptive patient once remarked, "I would like to go to O.T., and I would probably get something out of it, but once you start going, you have to go for life." In his experience, the only persons who ever finished O.T. were those who left the treatment setting or those who died. You start setting treatment priorities right now by prioritizing your patient's problems. Two decisions need to be made: which problems are appropriate for your intervention, and in what order you will work on them.

At this point you have already defined the problems using an O.T. frame of reference; thus it can be assumed you have written problems that are theoretically amenable to O.T. treatment. These problems will differ depending on the frame of reference you are using (Tables 2-2 through 2-5). The next step is to determine which of these problems are reasonable to address given the resources and constraints of your treatment facility. For instance, both the anticipated length of the patient's stay and the intensity of his symptoms have an impact on problem selection. A stay of two weeks, mostly spent in the management of acute symptoms, implies the treatment of different problems than an indeterminate stay in a day-treatment program. Building job habits is neither effective nor appropriate when your patient is acutely symptomatic, but may be very appropriate when the symptoms are under control.

Sometimes difficult choices must be made. Limiting the problems you tackle at one time increases your chances of successful outcomes. Fortunately, occupational therapists do not work in a vacuum; other professionals and agencies are usually involved with the patient. So, although you cannot provide all the treatment your patient needs yourself, you can coordinate the treatment and follow-up with other occupational therapists in community agencies.

The following criteria, paraphrased from Bloom and Fischer, can be used to prioritize your patient's problems [16].

1. Does the patient want to start with this problem? Is it the one about which he is the most concerned?
2. Does this problem have the greatest likelihood of being resolved?
3. Is the problem relatively concrete and specific?
4. Can you work with the problem within your given resources?
5. If the problem is not handled, does it have the greatest likelihood of producing the most negative consequences?
6. Does this problem need to be tackled before other problems can be addressed?
7. Will work on the problem result in tangible, observable changes in the patient, thereby increasing his motivation to address other problems?

Your Turn

Write each of the following concerns as a problem with at least two specific indicators (you will have to make up details). These concerns are stated as generic concepts. Use a frame of reference for each concern and practice writing problems and indicators using the correct terminology for that frame of reference. (Review Tables 2-2 through 2-5 for assistance.) To check the specificity, subject your problems and indicators to the clarity, observability, and reification tests.

Concern	Problem	Indicators
Not assertive	Does not express opinions	Has never expressed preferences for leisure activities to spouse (e.g., movie, restaurant)
		Self-reported high degree of discomfort in verbal groups
Low self-esteem		
Disoriented		
Has lots of free time		

Identifying Strengths

Early in your professional training, you were probably introduced to O.T.'s philosophy of treating the whole person [79,89,104]. Inherent in this philosophy is identifying and addressing the patient's strengths as well as his problems. Theoretically, we know that identifying strengths is important. In day-to-day practice, however, it is easy to become preoccupied with the patient's problems, as they are the usual reason for referral to O.T. and, therefore, the focus of your treatment. Rogers suggests, however, that lack of attention to strengths results in a skewed perception of your patient in which you are likely to overestimate his problems and underestimate his abilities [92]. Identifying strengths not only provides a more accurate picture of your patient's functioning, but also uncovers potential resources. Your patient can use his strengths to cope with, adapt to, compensate for, or overcome his problems. Take the time to identify them now. They will be needed when you write the goals and determine treatment methods.

Your Turn

Copy the problems and indicators you wrote for the last exercise in the spaces below. Add at least one strength for each problem (you will need to supply some details).

Problem	Indicators	Strengths
Does not express opinions	Has never expressed preferences for leisure activities to spouse (e.g., movie or restaurant)	Has opinions and desires to express them
	Self-reported high degree of discomfort in verbal groups	Self-reported dissatisfaction with current level of assertiveness

Sources of Error

Despite our best intentions, sometimes we make errors in identifying problems. The two major sources of therapist error are measurement error and therapist bias.

Measurement Error

Measurement error results from improper use of instruments, misinterpretation of the results, or both. Failure to use a standardized instrument as instructed by the protocol, use for nonendorsed purposes and populations, and use of only part of the instrument invalidate the results. The point is, you do not really know how much these variations affect the results, so they must be interpreted with the same limitations as nonstandardized instruments.

Because the standardization data for most O.T. instruments is preliminary and somewhat limited, you must interpret the results with caution. No one knows enough at this point to make unequivocal, definitive statements. This does not mean you should be afraid to say anything. Obviously the more standardization data there is on an instrument, the more confidence you can place in the results. Multiple measurements also increase your confidence in the results. Until the instruments are developed further, your interpretations need to be presented in qualified terms. (See Chap. 4 for specific examples of wording.)

Therapist Bias

Recent research suggests that therapists are subject to several forms of personal bias that affect their clinical decisions. First, therapists tend to overestimate the patient's pathology [29]. Frequently there is a discrepancy between the therapist's and the patient's perception of the nature and severity of his problems [92,109]. Therapists often tend to attribute the patient's problems to internal causes rather than to external factors [12,92]. They are thus more likely to attribute a patient's difficulty getting along with roommates to his lack of assertiveness than to the possibility of an unreasonable living situation. Of course, therapists generally have a better picture of the patient than of his environment. "Nevertheless, it should be recognized that our 'clinic-bound' view of the patient may lead us to ignore and underestimate impediments . . . residing in the environment" [92, p. 612]. Looking at the patient in his environment is part of O.T.'s domain of concern for all frames of reference, and it can be one area in which O.T. makes a unique contribution in psychiatric treatment.

Additionally, therapists seem to rate their patient's behavior as significantly more pathologic than do the patients themselves. This discrepancy is often explained as the patient's denial of his symptoms or disorder. Certainly psychiatric disorders can create denial and lack of awareness of the severity of symptoms. On the other hand, some studies suggest that the patient's perceptions (of treatment effectiveness, at least) are more highly correlated with independent measures of successful outcome of therapy than are the therapist's perceptions [109]. Disregarding the patient's perceptions of the severity of his symptoms not only creates errors, but it also damages the therapeutic relationship.

A third source of therapist bias results from the perceived interpersonal attractiveness of the patient [31,92,109]. Patients who are liked by the therapist frequently receive more help. Inexperienced clinicians often find helpless, dependent patient behaviors reinforcing to their own feelings of helping, and these behaviors probably result in increased patient likableness. With experience, however, these same patient behaviors are more often perceived as negative by the clinician. Patients are then seen as weak, apathetic, and powerless, and therapists express more negativity about the patient's motivation for change [31].

When therapists become pessimistic about the effects of their work, they become tense, introverted, and withdrawn from their patients, a condition often described as burnout. Not only are they more prone to errors, but they also frequently become dissatisfied with their jobs and careers.

What can be done? Fehrenback and O'Leary suggest using the following strategies to minimize therapist bias [31]. Make it a habit to identify the patient's strengths as well as his problems to balance your overall impression of his functioning. If you are working with a patient you dislike, look for areas in which the two of you are similar. Finding commonalities will increase his likability to you and your investment in him. You may be shocked to read that there will be some patients you may not like; after all, is that acceptable? Regardless of our intent to care for everyone equally, there will be some patients who are very difficult to like. Because liking the patient is associated with more effective treatment [110], adopting strategies to minimize the errors resulting from hidden biases seems preferable to denying that the problem exists. When identifying problems, present evidence (to yourself) both for and against the problem. That is, what evidence do you have that indicates this issue is a problem for your patient, and what evidence do you have that indicates it is not a problem? Looking equally at both sides of the picture will help reduce your tendency to find problems just because you are looking for them. Finally, do not neglect the role of your patient's environment in his current functioning. Identification of all contributing factors guides your treatment efforts; helping the patient change his environment may supersede helping him change himself.

Therapist error can be minimized by developing rigorous clinical habits and vigilant self-monitoring. Although you are inexperienced at this point, you are also less prone to therapist error because you are conscious (sometimes painfully so) of everything you are doing. Converting that self-consciousness into conscientiousness is the best defense for minimizing the chances of making errors.

Your Turn

Therapist error is rarely intentional; we may not even be aware when it occurs. Gaining awareness of our own biases helps prevent us from inadvertently acting on them and making errors. The following questions are meant to stimulate your thinking. The issue here is not whether having biases is right or wrong, but rather to identify them so they do not affect our clinical decisions. Although these questions apply to work in all areas of O.T., for now confine your answers to psychiatry.

1. At this point, what type of patient characteristics, behaviors, or problems would it be easiest for you to work with?

Reasons?

2. At this point, what type of patient characteristics, behaviors, or problems would it be difficult for you to work with?

Reasons?

3. Suppose your patient disagreed with you about either the nature or severity of his problems. How would you handle this situation?

4. At this point, which form(s) of therapist error are you most likely to exhibit?

Strategy for prevention?

Share your thoughts with your classmates. You will not only broaden your perspectives, but you will also be starting a good habit of seeking support from professional colleagues.

Summary
This section addressed the final step of the assessment process: synthesis of all the information you have collected and identification of your patient's problems and strengths. You have gone through the whole process on paper, now it is time to try it out in clinical practice.

Right now?
Right here?
Me?
*Sondra Anice Barnes**

This chapter has introduced you to the assessment process—from screening to identifying the patient's problems and problem indicators. Now it is time to try it with a patient. Starting with screening, proceed step by step through the assessment process. The forms you need are reprinted for your convenience. Pay particular attention to any question or difficulty you have along the way; these are clues that you need more work in those areas.

The patient, presumably, has already been referred to O.T. Use the following chart to help orient yourself to the procedures your facility has for handling referrals.

Referrals

Is a referral necessary to deliver O.T. services?

Who is the source of referrals? (Specific names help the most.)

What is the process for receiving referrals?

Where are the referrals put?

Who processes the doctor's orders?

How do you bring the need for the referral to the doctor's attention?

Is the process usually expedient?

Is there any way to speed up the process if there are delays?

Within what time frame do you need to respond to a referral?

How are weekend referrals handled?

Where is the note written in the chart?

What is the suggested format for responding to referral notes?

*From *Life Is The Way It Is* (copyright © 1978 by Brason-Sargar Publications, P.O. Box 872, Reseda, California 91335).

Notes to myself:

Chart Review

Next you are ready to complete the chart review. Make sure to note any term, medication, or abbreviation you are unfamiliar with so you can look it up later.

Name: Date:

Physician: Diagnosis:

Medications: Precautions:

Presenting problems:

Mental status:

History of present illness:

Other:

Notes to myself:

Selecting a Frame of Reference

Based on the information you have collected so far about both the patient and the treatment facility, select a frame of reference.

Frame of reference:

Basis for the selection:

Notes to myself:

Interview and Performance Measure

Using the principles of the frame of reference you selected and your knowledge of the patient, select the content and format for both the interview and the performance measure.

Interview

1. Content:

2. Format:

Performance measure

1. Content:

2. Format:

Basis for selection:

Notes to myself:

Review the principles of interviewing in Chap. 1 if you need a booster; then it is time to conduct your interview and performance measure.

When you have completed these steps, take a few minutes to review your performance. This interview self-evaluation was also used in Chap. 1. Compare your performance on this interview with the one you did in the last chapter. Was it different?

Interview Self-Evaluation

Attending skills	Good	Needs work
1. Preparation of the subject: your introduction of the purpose of the interview	——	——
2. Preparation of the setting: physical surroundings private and conducive	——	——
3. Attending actions: your positioning, eye contact, and use of back channels	——	——
4. Nurturing: use of any nurturing action	——	——
5. Avoidance of listening blocks or distortions	——	——
6. Observation skills: tone of voice, nonverbal expression, and congruence	——	——
7. Match of listening level to the level required	——	——
8. Appropriate use of social chitchat	——	——
9. Paraphrasing:		
Appropriate levels	——	——
Correct sequence	——	——
10. Questions:		
Use of open and closed questions	——	——
Use of secondary questions	——	——
Avoidance of double, directed, or why questions	——	——

11. Use of feedback   ____   ____
12. Progression of the interview: moving from opening, to
    body, to closing   ____   ____

Performance Measure Self-Evaluation

How did the session go?

Was the performance measure appropriate?

  If no, what would have been better?

Notes to myself:

Preliminary Data Synthesis

Now you are at the point of deciding whether you have enough information to proceed with stating problems, or whether you need to conduct additional evaluations. If you think you can write problems and indicators at this point, skip the next section and proceed directly with writing problems. If you need to do additional evaluations, select the instruments you will use.

Notes to myself:

Instrument Selection

Use the following questions to help guide your choice of evaluation instruments.

1. Identify the patient's specific problem areas that require further evaluation:

2. Of the categories of instruments, which best measure this area of function for your patient?

3. Basis for that opinion:

4. Of the categories of instruments you identified, which specific instruments are recommended by the frame of reference you are using with this patient?

5. What are the practical constraints of your treatment facility that have an impact on the instrument you select?

6. State which instrument(s) you will use to evaluate the patient further?

7. Basis for that selection:

Notes to myself:

Evaluation

Now that you have selected the evaluation instruments, you can administer them. When done, take a few minutes to review how the session(s) went.

Evaluation Instrument Self-Evaluation

Were the instruments I used appropriate?

Why or why not?

Were the goals of the session met?

What helped or hindered reaching the goals?

What did I do that was effective? (You want to make sure you can do it again):

What did I do that was not effective? (You want to make sure you do not do it again):

Notes to myself:

Data Synthesis and Interpretation

The final step is to synthesize the information you have and produce a list of the patient's problems, problem indicators, and strengths. Remember that problems need to be stated as specifically as possible. Specificity means the problems are clear, observable, and not reified. Write at least two problem indicators for each problem.

Indicators should be information from your screening or evaluation that specifically states how this concern is a problem for your patient. After each indicator, state the source of the data (interview, performance measure, instrument). Finally, do not forget to list his strengths. Try to find a strength for each problem you list. For now, do not worry about prioritizing the problems; concentrate on writing specific problems and indicators.

Problem	Indicators	Strengths

Notes to myself:

Finally, prioritize the problems. They should be ranked with number 1 assigned to the most important problem (the one that has the most affirmative answers to the following questions).

1. Does the patient want to start with this problem? Is it the one about which he is the most concerned?
2. Does this problem have the greatest likelihood of being resolved?
3. Is the problem relatively concrete and specific?
4. Can you treat the problem within your given resources?
5. If the problem is not handled, does it have the greatest likelihood of producing the most negative consequences?
6. Does this problem need to be tackled before other problems can be addressed?
7. Will work on the problem result in tangible, observable changes in the patient, thereby increasing his motivation to address other problems?

Notes to myself:

Congratulations! You have successfully completed the assessment process and you are ready to move on to treatment planning. Do not get discouraged if this seemed to take you a while to complete. With continued experience and clinical growth, this process of organizing information will become integrated and almost second nature.

1. Allen, C. K. Independence through activity: The practice of occupational therapy (psychiatry). *Am. J. Occup. Ther.* 36:731, 1982.

2. Allen, C. K. *Occupational Therapy for Psychiatric Diseases: Measurement and Management of Cognitive Disabilities.* Boston: Little, Brown, 1985.

3. American Occupational Therapy Association. Uniform occupational therapy evaluation checklist. *Am. J. Occup. Ther.* 35:817, 1981.

4. American Psychiatric Association. APA Standards for Educational and Psychological Tests and Manuals. In D. N. Jackson and S. Messick (eds.), *Problems in Human Assessment.* New York: McGraw-Hill, 1978.

5. American Psychiatric Association. *Diagnostic and Statistical Manual of Mental Disorders* (3rd ed.). Washington, DC: American Psychiatric Association, 1980.

5a. Ayers, A. J. *Sensory Integration and Learning Disorders.* Los Angeles: Western Psychological Services, 1972.

6. Ayers, A. J. *Southern California Sensory Integration Tests Manual.* Los Angeles: Western Psychological Services, 1972.

7. Ayers, A. J. *Sensory Integration and The Child.* Los Angeles: Western Psychological Services, 1979.

8. Barlow, D. H., Hayes, S. C., and Nelson, R. O. *The Scientist Practioner: Research and Accountability in Clinical and Educational Settings.* New York: Pergamon, 1984.

9. Barris, R. Environmental interactions: An extension of the model of occupation. *Am. J. Occup. Ther.* 36:637, 1982.

10. Barris, R., Kielhofner, G., and Watts, J. H. *Psychosocial Occupational Therapy: Practice in a Pluralistic Arena.* Laurel, MD: Ramsco, 1983.

11. Barris, R., Oakley, F., and Kielhofner, G. The Role Checklist. *Occup. Ther. J. Res.* 6:157, 1986.

12. Batson, C. D., O'Quinn, K., and Pych, V. An Attribution Theory Analysis of Trained Helpers' Inferences About Clients' Needs. In T. A. Wills (ed.), *Basic Processes in Helping Relationships.* New York: Academic, 1982.

13. Beard, J. G., and Ragheb, M. G. Measuring leisure satisfaction. *J. Leisure Res.* 12:20, 1980.

14. Benson, J., and Clark, F. A guide for instrument development and validation. *Am. J. Occup. Ther.* 36:789, 1982.

15. Black, M. M. Adolescent role assessment. *Am. J. Occup. Ther.* 30:73, 1976.

16. Bloom, M., and Fischer, J. *Evaluating Practice: Guidelines for the Accountable Professional.* Englewood Cliffs, NJ: Prentice-Hall, 1982.

17. Bloomer, J., and Williams, S. *Bay Area Functional Performance Evaluation (BaFPE): Task Oriented Assessment and Social Interaction Scale Manual.* San Francisco: USCF, 1979.

18. Bloomer, J., and Williams, S. The Bay Area Functional Performance Evaluation. In B. J. Hemphill (ed.), *The Evaluative Process in Psychiatric Occupational Therapy.* Thorofare, NJ: Slack, 1982.

19. Bloomer, J., and Williams, S. The Revised Bay Areas Functional Performance Evaluation. Unpublished data, 1985.

20. Boker, A. M. Assessment: The keystone of treatment planning. *Occup. Ther. Health Care* 1:25, 1984.

21. Brayman, S. J., et al. Comprehensive occupational therapy evaluation scale. *Am. J. Occup. Ther.* 30:94, 1976.

22. Brayman, S. J., and Kirby, T. The Comprehensive Occupational Therapy Evaluation. In B. J. Hemphill (ed.), *The Evaluative Process in Psychiatric Occupational Therapy.* Thorofare, NJ: Slack, 1982.

23. Briggs, A. K., et al. *Case Simulations in Psychosocial Occupational Therapy.* Philadelphia: Davis, 1979.

24. Buck, R. E., and Provancher, M. A. Magazine picture collages as an evaluation technique. *Am. J. Occup. Ther.* 26:36, 1972.

25. Clark, E. N., and Peters, M. Scorable Self Care Evaluation Manual. Thorofare, NJ: Slack, 1984.

26. Clark, P. N. Human development through occupation: Theoretical frameworks in contemporary occupational therapy practice, Part 1. *Am. J. Occup. Ther.* 33:305, 1979.

27. Clark, P. N. Human development through occupation: A philosophy and conceptual model for practice, Part 2. *Am. J. Occup. Ther.* 33:577, 1979.

28. Cynkin, S. *Occupational Therapy: Toward Health Through Activities.* Boston: Little, Brown, 1979.

29. Dawes, R. M. The Value of Being Explicit When Making Clinical Decisions. In T. A. Wills (ed.), *Basic Processes in Helping Relationships.* New York: Academic, 1982.

30. Ethridge, D. A. Pre-vocational assessment of rehabilitation potential. *Am. J. Occup. Ther.* 23:161, 1968.

31. Fehrenback, P. A., and O'Leary, M. R. Interpersonal Attraction and Treatment Decisions in Inpatient and Outpatient Settings. In T. A. Wills (ed.), *Basic Processes in Helping Relationships.* New York: Academic, 1982.

32. Fidler, G. S. From crafts to competency. *Am. J. Occup. Ther.* 35:567, 1981.

33. Fidler, G. S. The Lifestyle Performance Profile: An Organizing Frame. In B. J. Hemphill (ed.), *The Evaluative Process in Psychiatric Occupational Therapy.* Thorofare, NJ: Slack, 1982.

34. Fidler, G. S. *Design of Rehabilitation Services in Psychiatric Hospital Settings.* Laurel, MD: Ramsco, 1984.

35. Fidler, G. S., and Fidler, J. W. *Occupational Therapy: A Communication Process in Psychiatry.* New York: Macmillan, 1963.

36. Fidler, G. S., and Fidler, J. W. Doing and becoming: Purposeful action and self actualization. *Am. J. Occup. Ther.* 32:305, 1978.

37. Fine, S. *Occupational Therapy: The Role of Rehabilitation and Purposeful Activity in Mental Health.* Rockville, MD: American Occupational Therapy Association, 1983.

38. Florey, L. L., and Michelman, S. M. Occupational role history: A screening tool for psychiatric occupational therapy. *Am. J. Occup. Ther.* 36:301, 1982.

39. Frankl, V. E. *Man's Search for Meaning.* New York: Simon and Schuster, 1963.

40. Garfield, S. T. *Psychotherapy: An Eclectic Approach.* New York: Wiley, 1980.

41. Good-Ellis, M., et al. *Role Activity Performance Scale.* Unpublished data, 1985.

42. Harlan, B. Determining the reliability of the occupational role history. Virginia Commonwealth University Master's Thesis, 1983.

43. Hasselkus, B. R., and Safrit, M. J. Measurement in occupational therapy. *Am. J. Occup. Ther.* 30:429, 1976.

44. Haynes, S. N. Behavioral Assessment. In M. Hernsen, A. E. Kazdin, and A. S. Bellack (eds.), *The Clinical Psychology Handbook.* New York: Pergamon, 1983.

45. Hemphill, B. J. Mental health evaluations used in occupational therapy. *Am. J. Occup. Ther.* 34:721, 1980.

46. Hemphill, B. J. *Training Manual for the B. H. Battery.* Thorofare, NJ: Slack, 1982.

47. Hemphill, B. J. The BH Battery. In B. J. Hemphill (ed.), *The Evaluative Process in Psychiatric Occupational Therapy.* Thorofare, NJ: Slack, 1982.

48. Hemphill, B. J. The Evaluative Process. In B. J. Hemphill (ed.), *The Evaluative Process In Psychiatric Occupational Therapy.* Thorofare, NJ: Slack, 1982.

49. Hinojosa, J., et al. Roles and functions of the occupational therapist in the treatment of sensory integrative dysfunction. *Am. J. Occup. Ther.* 36:833, 1982.

50. Holland, J. L. *The Self-Directed Search Manual.* Palo Alto, CA: Consulting Psychologists, 1979.

51. Howe, M. C., and Briggs, A. K. Ecological systems model for occupational therapy. *Am. J. Occup. Ther.* 36:322, 1982.

52. Hsu, Y. T., and Nelson, D. L. Adult performance on the Southern California kinesthesis and tactile perception tests. *Am. J. Occup. Ther.* 35:788, 1981.

53. Huss, A. J. From kinesiology to adaptation. *Am. J. Occup. Ther.* 35:574, 1981.

54. Kaplan, K. Short-term assessment: The need and a response. *Occup. Ther. Ment. Health* 4:29, 1984.

55. Kazdin, A. E. Treatment Research: The Investigation and Evaluation of Psychotherapy. In M. Hersen, A. E. Kazdin, and A. S. Bellack (eds.), *The Clinical Psychology Handbook.* New York: Pergamon, 1983.

56. Kielhofner, G. *Health Through Occupation: Theory and Practice in Occupational Therapy.* Philadelphia: Davis, 1983.

57. Kielhofner, G. (ed.) *A Model of Human Occupation: Theory and Application.* Baltimore: Williams & Wilkins, 1985.

58. Kielhofner, G., and Barris, R. Mental health occupational therapy: Trends in literature and practice. *Occup. Ther. Ment. Health* 4:35, 1984.

59. Kielhofner, G., and Burke, J. P. A model of human occupation, Part 1: Conceptual framework and content. *Am. J. Occup. Ther.* 34:572, 1980.

60. Kielhofner, G., Burke, J. P., and Igi, C. H. A model of human occupation, Part 4: Assessment and intervention. *Am. J. Occup. Ther.* 34:777, 1980.

61. King, L. J. A sensory integrative approach to schizophrenia. *Am. J. Occup. Ther.* 28:529, 1974.

62. King, L. J. Notes on Assessment: Unpublished data, 1975.

63. King, L. J. Eleanor Clarke Slagle Lectureship, 1978—Towards a science of adaptive responses. *Am. J. Occup. Ther.* 32:429, 1978.

64. King, L. J. The Person Symbol As an Assessment Tool. In B. J. Hemphill (ed.), *The Evaluative Process in Psychiatric Occupational Therapy.* Thorofare, NJ: Slack, 1982.

64a. King, L. J. Occupational Therapy and Neuropsychiatry. *Occup. Ther. Ment. Health* 3:1, 1983.

65. Lambert, M. J. Introduction to Assessment in Psychotherapy Outcome: Historical Perspectives and Current Issues. In M. J. Lambert, E. R. Christensen, and S. S. DeJulio (eds.), *The Assessment of Psychotherapy Outcome.* New York: Wiley, 1983.

66. Lerner, C. The Magazine Picture Collage. In B. J. Hemphill (ed.), *The Evaluative Process in Psychiatric Occupational Therapy.* Thorofare, NJ: Slack, 1982.

67. Lerner, C., and Ross, G. The magazine picture collage: Development of an objective scoring system. *Am. J. Occup. Ther.* 31:156, 1977.

68. Llorens, L. L. *Appliation of a Developmental Theory for Health and Rehabilitation.* Rockville, MD: American Occupational Therapy Association, 1976.

69. Llorens, L. L. Theoretical conceptualizations of occupational therapy: 1960–1982. *Occup. Ther. Ment. Health* 4:1, 1984.

70. Llorens, L. L., and Gillette, N. P. The challenge for research in a practice profession. *Am. J. Occup. Ther.* 39:143, 1985.

71. Mack, W., Lindquist, J. E., and Parham, L. D. A synthesis of occupational behavior and sensory integration concepts in theory and practice, Part 1: Theoretical foundations. *Am. J. Occup. Ther.* 36:365, 1982.

72. Mack, W., Lindquist, J. E., and Parham, L. D. A synthesis of occupational behavior and sensory integration concepts in theory and practice, Part 2: Clinical applications. *Am. J. Occup. Ther.* 36:433, 1982.

73. Matsutsuyu, J. S. The interest check list. *Am. J. Occup. Ther.* 23:323, 1969.

74. Maurer, P., et al. Hierarchy of competencies relating to the use of standardized instruments and evaluation techniques by occupational therapists. *Am. J. Occup. Ther.* 38:803, 1984.

75. McGourty, L. K. *Kohlman Evaluation of Living Skills* (2nd ed.). Seattle: KELS Research, 1979.

76. Moorhead, L. The occupational history. *Am. J. Occup. Ther.* 23:329, 1969.

77. Mosey, A. C. *Three Frames of Reference for Mental Health.* Thorofare, NJ: Slack, 1970.

78. Mosey, A. C. An alternative: The biopsychosocial model. *Am. J. Occup. Ther.* 28:137, 1974.

79. Mosey, A. C. *Occupational Therapy: Configuration of a Profession.* New York: Raven, 1981.

80. Mosey, A. C. A monistic or a pluralistic approach to professional identity? *Am. J. Occup. Ther.* 39:504, 1985.

81. Moyer, E. A. A review of initial assessments used by occupational therapists in mental health settings. *Occup. Ther. Health Care* 1:33, 1984.

81a. Nelville, A. The model of human occupation and depression. *Mental Health Special Interest Section Newsletter* 8:1, 1985.

82. Newman, F. L. Therapist's Evaluation of Psychotherapy. In M. J. Lambert, E. R. Christensen, and S. S. DeJulio (eds.), *The Assessment of Psychotherapy Outcome.* New York: Wiley, 1983.

83. Oakley, F., Kielhofner, G., and Barris, R. An occupational therapy approach to assessing psychiatric patients' adaptive functioning. *Am. J. Occup. Ther.* 39:147, 1985.

84. Ostrow, P. C., and Kuntavanish, A. A. Improving the utilization of occupational therapy: A quality assurance study. *Am. J. Occup. Ther.* 37:388, 1983.

85. Parker, T. *Rules of Thumb.* Boston: Houghton Mifflin, 1983.

86. Peterson, P., and Wikoff, R. L. The performance of adult males on the Southern California figure-ground visual perception test. *Am. J. Occup. Ther.* 37:554: 1983.

87. Peterson, P., Goar, D., and Van Deusen, J. Performance of female adults on the Southern California visual figure-ground perception test. *Am. J. Occup. Ther.* 39:525, 1985.

88. Posthuma, B. W. Sensory integration in mental health: Dialogue with Lorna Jean King. *Occup. Ther. Ment. Health* 3:1, 1983.

89. Reed, K. L., and Sanderson, S. R. *Concepts of Occupational Therapy* (2nd ed.). Baltimore: Williams & Wilkins, 1983.

90. Reilly, M. A psychiatric occupational therapy program as a teaching model. *Am. J. Occup. Ther.* 20:61, 1966.

91. Reker, G. T., and Peacock, E. J. The life attitude profile (LAP): A multidimensional instrument for assessing attitudes towards life. *Can. J. Behav. Sci./Rev. Can. Sci. Comp.* 13:264, 1981.

92. Rogers, J. C. Eleanor Clarke Slagle Lectureship, 1983—Clinical Reasoning: The ethics, science, and art. *Am. J. Occup. Ther.* 37:601, 1983.

93. Rogers, C. R., and Skinner, B. F. Some Issues Concerning the Control of Human Behavior. In D. L. Avila, A. W. Combs, and W. W. Purkey (eds.), *The Helping Relationship Sourcebook.* Boston: Allyn and Bacon, 1973.

94. Rogers, J. C., Weinstein, J. M., and Figone, J. J. The interest checklist: An empirical assessment. *Am. J. Occup. Ther.* 32:628, 1978.

95. Scardina, V. From pegboards to integration. *Am. J. Occup. Ther.* 35:581, 1981.

95a. Schroeder, C. V., and Herberg, A. K. *Adult Sensory Integration Treatment Manual.* Kailua, HA: Schroeder, 1981.

96. Schroeder, C. V., et al. *SBC Adult Psychiatric Sensory Integration Evaluation Manual.* La Jolla, CA: SBC Research Associates, 1978.

97. Schroeder, C. V., et al. The Adult Psychiatric Sensory Integration Evaluation. In B. J. Hemphill (ed.), *The Evaluative Process in Psychiatric Occupational Therapy.* Thorofare, NJ: Slack, 1982.

98. Schulman, E. *Intervention in Human Services.* New York: Mosby, 1974.

99. Seig, K. W. Applying the behavioral model to the occupational therapy model. *Am. J. Occup. Ther.* 28:421, 1974.

100. Shannon, P. D. The derailment of occupational therapy. *Am. J. Occup. Ther.* 31:229, 1977.

101. Stein, F. A current review of the behavioral frame of reference and its application to occupational therapy. *Occup. Ther. Ment. Health* 2:35, 1982.

102. Swonger, A. K., and Constantine, L. L. *Drugs and Therapy: A Handbook of Psychotropic Drugs.* Boston: Little, Brown, 1983.

103. Taube, C. A., et al. Prospective payment and psychiatric discharges from general hospitals with and without psychiatric units. *Hosp. Community Psychiatry* 36:754, 1985.

104. Tiffany, E. G. Psychiatry and Mental Health. In H. L. Hopkins and H. D. Smith (eds.), *Willard and Spackman's Occupational Therapy* (5th ed.). New York: Lippincott, 1978.

105. Utley, E. R. Sensory Integrative Theory in Psychiatry. Unpublished data, 1984.

106. Van Dalen, D. B. *Understanding Educational Research: An Introduction* (3rd ed.). New York: McGraw-Hill, 1973.

107. Watts, J. H., et al. The Assessment of Occupational Functioning: Development of a Screening Instrument for Use in Long Term Care Facilities. *Am. J. Occup. Ther.* 40:231, 1986.

108. Weiner, I. B. Theoretical Foundations of Clinical Psychology. In M. Hersen, A. E. Kazdin, and A. S. Bellack (eds.), *The Clinical Psychology Handbook.* New York: Pergamon, 1983.

109. Wills, T. A. Directions for Research on Helping Relationships. In T. A. Wills (ed.), *Basic Processes in Helping Relationships.* New York: Academic, 1982.

110. Wills, T. A. Nonspecific Factors in Helping Relationships. In T. A. Wills (ed.), *Basic Processes in Helping Relationships.* New York: Academic, 1982.

"Please do not be alarmed," it said, "by anything you see or hear around you. . . . We will be restoring normality just as soon as we are sure what is normal anyway."

Douglas Adams
Hitchhiker's Guide to the Galaxy

Jo Rabson felt pleased with herself. She had completed Mr. Casey's screening and had selected and administered an evaluation instrument. She seemed to have voluminous data, but with persistence (something most O.T. students possess), she identified several problems and their indicators, prioritized them, noted Mr. Casey's strengths, and was ready to begin treatment. Somewhat concerned with how long the process took her, Jo wondered how she would manage with more than one patient. Heartened by her supervisor's reassurance that she would become more efficient with experience, she turned her attention to Mr. Casey's treatment. What should she have him do? Suppose he did not want to do anything she could find in the O.T. clinic? Could she convince him to do something he did not want to do? Should she even try? To her dismay, she saw lots of craft supplies in the O.T. clinic. While in school, Jo had not felt particularly comfortable with the idea of using crafts, and she felt even less comfortable now that she stood face to face with a cupboard full of leather belts and tile trivets. What if Mr. Casey wanted just to sit and talk? Should she let him? What purpose would it serve?

In her continuing adventures as an affiliating O.T. student, Jo raises several pertinent questions about the treatment process. Anxious to get started, Jo jumped from problem identification to selecting an activity to carry out the treatment, missing the critical intermediate step of setting goals. Without determining the goals and objectives of treatment, Jo will not know what she is trying to accomplish or how to go about it. Picking an activity (the method) before identifying the goal is a little like a doctor walking into the pharmacy and saying, "Gee, I wonder what I'll use today." He might serendipitously stumble across the right medication and its proper dose, but would you risk it? Professional responsibility to deliver the services promised dictates that one selects treatment methods based on more than chance.

This chapter addresses the last three phases of the treatment process:

1. *Treatment planning.* Identify goals, objectives, and methods of treatment.
2. *Treatment implementation.* Begin treatment, evaluate results, and revise plan as needed.
3. *Termination of treatment.* Discontinue O.T. when treatment is completed.

Your Turn
The terminology used in writing goals is confusing. In some instances, the terms *goal* and *objective* are used interchangeably; in other instances, they mean different things. Based on your current knowledge, define and give an example of each of the following terms. When you finish working through this chapter, you can review your definitions and revise them as necessary.

Term	*Definition*	*Example*
Goal		
Objective		
Performance		

Criterion

Condition

Method

Role of Theory

When you helped me,
you did it FOR me
because you knew
I couldn't do it.

When you assisted me,
you allowed ME to do it
because you knew
I could do it.
*Sondra Anice Barnes**

Treatment of psychiatric dysfunction is both challenging and exciting. Given that the treatment possibilities are extensive and often vary with each therapist, clinic, and frame of reference, how do you decide what is the best way to help each patient? As with interviews and assessments, the theoretic base of each frame of reference provides both a means of understanding what you see and corollary guidelines for treatment. The frames of reference do not provide a recipe for action, but they do articulate the basis from which you will make clinical decisions. Although at times you may be anxious to get into the nuts and bolts of treatment methods, a solid grounding in theory provides the foundation for your treatment-planning and implementation skills. Unless you understand the reasons behind various methods, your treatment will be, at best, serendipitous. To help get you started, the frames of reference discussed in this book are summarized in the following sections with an emphasis on treatment planning. This review is for comparison purposes only; further study of each is required before you proceed with actual treatment planning. Refer to the references at the end of the chapter for further study.

Functional Performance

The overall purpose of O.T. intervention is to improve the patient's performance of work, play, and self-maintenance tasks. Because performance in these areas is thought to involve five component systems (motor, psychologic, social, cognitive, and sensory integration), initial treatment efforts would be directed at dysfunction of these individual systems [18,19]. Dysfunction is thought to be remedied through learning new skills; thus, treatment is designed to encourage learning by doing [35]. "The nature of the occupational therapy setting, which effects active involvement in doing, provides a microcosm of life-work situations which can be seen and explored as they occur rather than in retrospect" [32, p. 45].

Skills must be learned both in their appropriate developmental sequence and in a way that will generalize to the patient's environment outside the treatment setting [18,19,32,79,80]. A variety of approaches for helping patients to learn by doing (also referred to as experiential learning) have been proposed, such as developmentally sequencing skill learning with educational taxonomies and using an educational-type structure with classes, teachers, students, and graduation to teach adaptive skills [67,105,108]. A wide range of activities are suggested as treatment methods. They are analyzed and selected for their cultural significance and age appropriateness for each patient. The activity's motor, sensory integrative, psychologic, cognitive, and social components are matched with the patient's problems, strengths, values, and learning readiness [32]. In this frame of reference, the therapist's role is to design a learning environment that fits the patient's needs and facilitates his learning of skills through active involvement in selected activities [18,19,32,80].

*From *Life Is The Way It Is* (copyright © 1978 by Brason-Sargar Publications, P.O. Box 872, Reseda, California 91335).

Sensory Integration

The overall purpose of O.T. intervention is to improve the patient's ability to interpret and respond to sensory information [11,43,55,100]. Because adequate sensory integration is thought to be a prerequisite for competent performance of daily life tasks, initial treatment efforts are directed at improving the patient's sensory processing dysfunction. This sensory processing dysfunction is thought to be remediated by reorganizing the patient's nervous system through the application of clear, repetitive sensory stimulation to the vestibular, proprioceptive, and tactile channels [43,90]. It is believed that improved sensory integrative functioning reduces symptoms and increases affect, self-esteem, ability to learn, verbalization, and self-confidence [58]. Sensory stimulation that elicits these adaptive responses must be developmentally sequenced, pleasurable, and subcortically integrated [55,59,72,73, 99]. Activities are analyzed for their sensory and motor properties and administered (usually self-directed) to elicit an adaptive response. "We could say that occupational therapy consists of structuring the surroundings, materials and especially the demands of the environment in such a way as to call forth a specific adaptive response" [56, p. 16]. In this frame of reference, the therapist's role is to plan and administer appropriate treatment, carefully monitor the patient for adverse facilitatory or inhibitory reactions during therapy, and maintain a pleasurable, nonthreatening atmosphere that encourages the patient's participation [43].

Model of Human Occupation

The overall purpose of O.T. intervention is to restore the organizational status of all systems: input, throughput, and feedback [8,51,52,85]. The throughput system is thought to consist of the volition, habituation, and performance subsystems, and initial treatment efforts are directed toward dysfunction of these subsystems [8,52]. The fit between the patient and his environment [7,8,52] is also considered in treatment planning. Cubie and Kaplan propose a case-analysis method for treatment planning that identifies 10 primary clinical questions with corresponding implications for treatment for each of the three subsystems [21]. Dysfunction is thought to be remediated by increasing the patient's awareness of his maladaptive occupational patterns through problem solving and planning and by offering him opportunities for involvement in activities (termed occupations) that allow him to practice adaptive patterns; thus dysfunction is remediated by promoting healthy functioning [8,52,54,84]. The treatment goals are set at the level of arousal, exploratory behavior, competence, or achievement that is required to encourage the patient's participation. Occupations are analyzed for their relationship to the three subsystems and matched with each patient's needs and cultural values. Patient involvement in productive occupations is seen as the fundamental basis of treatment. ". . . People can become competent and confident through what they do" [8, p. 281]. Occupations are thought to be healing: "that man, through the use of his hands as they are energized by mind and will, can influence the state of his own health" [93, p. 8]. In this frame of reference, the therapist's role is to analyze the organizational status of all systems, plan appropriate treatment, create meaning for the patient regarding his involvement in the occupation, and advocate for the patient by helping him to locate community resources, matching environmental demands to his capacities, and so forth [8].

Cognitive Disabilities

This frame of reference represents a major conceptual shift from the others that is especially relevant to treatment planning and implementation. The cognitive disabilities frame of reference does not make the patient the direct focus of intervention (as the other three do). Rather, it states that the overall purpose of O.T. intervention is to improve the patient's performance of routine tasks by changing (structuring, or adapting) the desired activity to facilitate his greater independence [1].

Psychiatric disease is thought to be divided into two categories: unstable and stable medical conditions. Both have implications for the type of O.T. services delivered. Unstable conditions, or acute mental diseases necessitate expectant, supportive, and palliative treatments. Stable medical conditions, or long-term disabilities, require compensations. Compensations can be biologic (alter the nervous system of the patient), psychologic (learn new skills to compensate for, or adapt to, deficits), or environmental (change the task to offset the defects in structure or function of the disabled person) [3]. The cognitive disabilities frame of reference focuses on the use of environmental compensations to help improve the patient's task behavior. ". . . In the verbal psychotherapies the common premise is that a person is unwilling to do a task but neuropathology would support the premise that a person is unable to do a task" [1, p. 734].

Another fundamental difference in the cognitive disabilities frame of reference is the location of the focus of O.T. intervention. It endorses changing the task rather than attempting to change the patient. Specific O.T. service objectives are identified for both treatment and compensation programs [3]. Selection of task content is left to the patient, as what may interest one person may not interest another. Whatever the task, the therapist can analyze and structure it to facilitate the patient's successful completion and greater independence in those routine tasks he wishes to do [1]. Properties of activities are analyzed and classified according to cognitive level of functioning. The therapist's role is to structure activities for the patient that will enable successful completion and facilitate greater independence [3].

Your Turn

By this point, you have become familiar with the basic principles of each of these four O.T. frames of reference. To help clarify what you know, fill in the following chart comparing these frames of reference with respect to treatment planning. (The frames of reference are coded as follows: FP = functional performance, SI = sensory integration, HO = human occupation, and CD = cognitive disabilities.)

	FP	SI	HO	CD
Definition of dysfunction and function				
Manner in which dysfunction is remediated				

Purpose of O.T. treatment

Type of O.T. treatment
  methods used

Focus of activity analysis

Role of therapist

How did you do? If you are missing some information or would like more indepth information about these frames of reference, check the references at the end of the chapter.

Goals and Objectives

If you're not sure where you're going, you're likely to end up someplace else.

Robert Mager

So far you have identified your patient's problems and strengths, and you are ready to start treatment. Before you start looking through the cupboards in the O.T. clinic for something that might work, you need to determine the intended outcome of your treatment (goal), the intermediate steps required to reach that goal (objectives), and the things you must do to reach the goal (methods).

The statement of the problem with specific indicators is a clear statement of *what is*. Goals are equally specific statements of *what should be*. In most instances, goals specify what changes are desired, direct the treatment, and provide standards to evaluate the outcome [12]. Goals provide direction for someone to do something, and, as such, are written for either the patient (outcome goals) or the therapist (process or service goals). The functional performance, sensory integration, and model of human occupation frames of reference use outcome goals because the patient is the direct focus of intervention. Process goals are used by the cognitive disabilities frame of reference because the task, not the patient, is the direct focus of intervention.

Outcome Goals

As the name implies, outcome goals indicate a behavior or outcome that is expected to result from treatment. In the 1960s, outcome goals were unfortunately called *behavioral goals* [74]. This term was easily misinterpreted to imply that therapists needed to use a behavioral approach, needed to be a behaviorist, or believed in behavior modification. In this context, however, *behavior* means a performance of some kind. As you learned in the last chapter, not all performances are overt or directly observable; some are covert and observable only to the patient. Regardless of whether the behaviors are overt or covert, the term *goals* describes the measurable outcome performances or behaviors expected to result from O.T. treatment.

Specificity vs "The Fuzzies"

Specificity is the ultimate pursuit in writing goals, but, as in all quests, obstacles block the path. The major obstacle to specificity is the tendency to lapse into vague abstractions, or, as Mager so aptly called them, the fuzzies [75]. Fuzzies are sneaky. They appear so often in our day-to-day conversations that we think we know what they mean. Yet, they do not specify exactly what the patient would be doing to indicate the goal had been reached. Goals such as *cope with stress*, *become aware of my feelings*, and *be socially appropriate* do not indicate what the patient would be doing when these goals are met; therefore, they are fuzzies. Fuzzies can be detected with Mager's "Hey, Dad!" test [75]. "Hey, Dad, look how I can cope with stress!" "Hey, Dad, look how I can be aware of my feelings!" "Hey, Dad, look how I can be socially appropriate!" Put in this way, they are easier to spot. Fuzzies are difficult because they sound "right" and generally have some meaning. Nevertheless, because they are vague, multiple interpretations occur. For instance, what would a person need to do to illustrate that he was coping with stress? Would he be eating three meals a day, sleeping eight hours a night, exercising regularly, communicating problems to his spouse without losing his temper, listening to a relaxation tape several times a week, going to yoga class, playing an aggressive sport to relieve tension, swimming 10 laps a day, sitting in the hot tub, or vacationing in the Bahamas? Unless you specify exactly what the patient is to achieve, you are left with only your hunches about his progress.

Avoiding fuzzies is easy when the goal represents an overt performance. Covert performances are more susceptible to vagueness, however, and you need to pay special attention to ferret out the fuzzies. You have already started this process. When you identified your patient's problems in the last chapter, you identified indicator behaviors that represented the covert performance. These indicators—usually expressed as an overt performance, self-monitoring report, or score on an instrument—can be translated into goals that pass the "Hey, Dad!" test [74,75]. For example:

Covert problem	Lack of assertiveness in making friends.
Indicator	Has not initiated contacts with friends in the past month.
	High degree of discomfort when speaking to new people.
	Low score on assertiveness inventory.
Covert goal	To improve assertiveness in making friends (fuzzy).
Outcome goals	Initiate two contacts each day with other patients (overt performance).
	Higher degree of comfort in speaking to new people (self-monitoring report).
	Higher score on assertiveness inventory (score on an instrument).

Are you still getting tricked by the fuzzies? The key question that identifies a fuzzy is, "What would the person be doing if this goal were being met." If the answer sounds silly, you know you have a fuzzy on your hands.

Your Turn
Check the fuzzy goals; that is, those that fail the "Hey, Dad!" test.

_____ 1. Increase coping skills
_____ 2. Take a shower, comb hair, brush teeth daily
_____ 3. Nonverbally express feelings of anger
_____ 4. Develop trust in others
_____ 5. Find volunteer job in two weeks
_____ 6. Communicate more effectively with others
_____ 7. Identify own strengths and weaknesses
_____ 8. Feel better about self
_____ 9. Learn one new leisure activity a month
_____ 10. Express feelings of frustration without losing temper

How did you do? Sometimes it is harder to recognize abstractions than you might think at first. In the following space, rewrite the fuzzies you identified into goals. Write at least two goals for each fuzzy, and specify whether it is an overt performance, a self-monitoring response, or a score on an instrument.

Problems and Goals

Goals are directly related to your patient's problems and indicators, as the goals represent what your patient would be doing if that problem were resolved. The following examples were taken from the lists of problems in the last chapter (p. 89). Each is related to a frame of reference (cognitive disabilities is addressed in a later section). Each problem refers to a different patient. (Key: FP = functional performance, SI = sensory integration, HO = model of human occupation.)

Problem	*Indicator*	*Goal*
Feels inferior to peers (FP)	Has not initiated contact with peers in past 6 months	Attend movie with peers two times in the next month
Impaired balance (SI)	Lost balance on Romberg in 4/4 trials	Able to perform Romberg with no difficulty and hold sharpened Romberg for 30 seconds
	Unable to hold sharpened Romberg for 10 seconds	
	Protective extension elicited in 3/4 trials	
Current role performance imbalance (HO)	Low satisfaction about current role performance	Higher rating of role performance satisfaction
	Discrepancy between valued roles and actual performance	Participate in two activities of valued role in next month

As these examples illustrate, goals are based on the patient's problem and its indicators. You may need one goal for each indicator, or you may be able to combine two indicators into one goal. Every problem identified on the problem list should have at least one corresponding goal or a reason why it is not being addressed at this time. See Chap. 4 for a suggested format for this documentation.

As commonalities can be expected in both the symptoms and the expected courses of disorders with similar diagnoses, some common problems can also be anticipated. Nevertheless, goals must be individualized, as each patient experiences his psychiatric disorder in a somewhat different manner. For instance, there could be many possible goals for the problem *feels inferior to peers. Attending a movie with peers two times in the next month* is only one possibility. Although it fits this patient, it may not be appropriate for another patient experiencing the same problem. The problem indicators reflect each patient's unique experiences and circumstances and naturally vary from patient to patient. Goals are therefore tailored to reflect these individual differences. As you may recall from Chap. 2, this patient's strengths included valuing friendships and having interests that could provide contact with peers (Table 2-2). These strengths were capitalized on in writing these goals.

Outcome goals are written to reflect the ultimate, terminal performance your patient is expected to achieve. What outcome level of performance can you reasonably expect of your patient in the amount of time you have to work with him? Will he return to his premorbid level of functioning, or will he have to learn to live with his limitations? These questions do not have easy answers. As professionals, occupational therapists strive to help patients function at their highest level possible [47,80,92,95,113]. Nevertheless, in view of the fact that not every patient can return to totally unimpaired functioning, O.T. services are generally divided into the following categories: prevention, treatment, rehabilitation, habilitation, and maintenance [57,80]. Each category has defined criteria for patient inclusion as well as specific expectations for outcome. The nature and course of the patient's disorder thus identify the type of treatment needed. Matching patients with these categories of treatment is clear for many physical illnesses. For instance, infants identified to be "at risk" may benefit from a preventive infant stimulation program, whereas children with neurologic processing dysfunction may benefit from sensory integration treatment programs. Stroke victims may benefit from rehabilitation programs, developmentally disabled persons from habilitation programs, and long-term-care geriatric residents from maintenance programs.

Matching patients with psychiatric disorders with appropriate treatment programs is less clear. Allen proposes using the acuity of the patient's disorder to determine appropriate O.T. services. When the patient is acutely ill and his disorder requires intensive medical management, appropriate types of O.T. services to offer include supportive, palliative, and expectant treatment. Compensatory O.T. services would be appropriate when the disorder has stabilized [3]. Each of these types of service has corresponding goals for treatment. Each psychiatric disorder is different and implies different expectations and hopes for return to unimpaired functioning. Consulting with other team members gives you some guidance about your patient's expected level of functioning and thus appropriate expected levels of performance.

Ultimately, your choice of outcome level of performance, whether a return to unimpaired functioning (cure) or an adaptation/coping strategy for residual problems (compensation), is based on your clinical judgment of the seriousness of the disorder and the length of time you have to work with your patient. With continued empirical studies of O.T.'s clinical effectiveness and theoretic frames of reference, occupational therapists should develop more expertise in predicting future impairment in the patient's functioning.

Your Turn

Write a corresponding goal for each of the following problems and problem indicators. The problems are associated with a particular frame of reference (see Tables 2-2 through 2-4). Use the postulates of that frame of reference to guide your selection of goal content. The purpose of this exercise is to give you practice in turning problems into goals. Aim for specificity, and double check your goals for fuzziness with the "Hey, Dad!" test. (Key: FP = functional performance, SI = sensory integration, and HO = model of human occupation.)

Problem	Indicators	Goals
Difficulty making decisions (FP)	Unable to choose between two tasks or two colors	
	Written notice from supervisor of performance decline	
Impaired bilateral coordination (SI)	Unable to draw Kephart circles in 3/3 trials	
	Does not discriminate between the right and left sides of the body	
Little interaction with other people outside of family (HO)	No role that requires involvement in social groups	
	No use of interests that include others	

Goal Components

Outcome goals have three components: performance (what is to be done), criterion (to what extent), and conditions (under what circumstances) [12,74]. Although goals may not always have the last two components, the performance must always be stated.

PERFORMANCE

By now, you are getting the idea that goals are written so the patient's performance, either overt or covert, can be measured. As Casey Stengel reportedly said, "If you don't know where you're going, you'll never know if you get there." Outcome goals use performances written from the patient's perspective, not the therapist's. *Providing purposeful activities to enhance self-esteem* is not an outcome goal because it states what the therapist will do, not the patient. In addition, the performance should be stated in positive terms (something the patient will do) rather than in negative terms (something he should not do). Lindsley refers to goals stated in negative terms (not striking out, not yelling) as the "dead man's error" [68]. These goals could be accomplished by a dead man; thus, they do not contribute to a hopeful atmosphere. Stating goals in positive terms helps to create the positive, expectant attitude of success that is needed to enhance the patient's commitment to treatment. Examples are

1. The patient tries new leisure interests.
2. The patient crosses midline.
3. The patient initiates contact with people.

The goals you wrote in the last exercise identified performances. Review them and ask yourself the following questions: Were they connected to the problem and problem indicators? Were they written from the patient's perspective—that is, stating what he would do? Were they stated in positive terms?

CRITERION

Criterion indicates the qualitative parameters of the performance. How well does the performance have to be done? Does it need to be done with speed? With accuracy? With quality? How many times? Criterion indicates to what degree the performance must be done before the goal is considered met. The criterion is determined from both a base line of data recording the patient's performance prior to treatment and input from the patient regarding desired levels of outcome. For instance, if a patient spent 4 hours out of bed each day before treatment, the criterion for the goal would be more than this amount and would also reflect the patient's preferences and responsibilities (e.g., job, family). Numeric criteria (e.g., 4/4 trials, 50% of the time, six times) are useful only when they are meaningful to the patient and not difficult to keep track of on a daily basis. Because human behavior is not an exact science, most criteria are set arbitrarily. Nevertheless, to be most effective, the criterion must represent an agreed-on estimation of what level of performance represents both progress and a reasonable challenge for your patient. Examples are

1. The patient tries *four new* leisure interests *in the next month.*
2. The patient crosses midline *on every trial.*
3. The patient *reports no discomfort* when initiating contact with people.

CONDITIONS

Along with the criterion, conditions provide the parameters for the performance. The conditions specify when, where, and with whom the performance should occur. Because not all problems occur in every situation and with every person with whom the patient interacts, the conditions specify under what circumstances the performance is expected to occur. If *inability to express needs without losing temper* occurred only on the job, then the conditions would specify that situation. If *discomfort in initiating contact with people* occurred primarily in social situations, the conditions would identify this specific problematic situation to address in treatment. Examples are

1. The patient tries four new leisure interests *involving other people* in the next month.
2. The patient crosses midline *on subcortical tasks* on every trial.
3. The patient reports no discomfort when initiating contact *with persons of the opposite sex.*

These three components—performance, criterion, and conditions—provide the format for writing outcome goals. Including these components in the goal increases its specificity and the chances that the goal can be achieved [12].

Your Turn

Rewrite the goals of the last exercise in the following space, and add both criteria and conditions. You need to speculate on these two parameters because you lack a base line of data and patient input. The purpose of this assignment is to increase your ability to write goals with all three components. Involving the patient in the treatment planning process helps provide the information you need to identify the performance, criterion, and conditions of the goal. For now, concentrate on the process, not the accuracy of the content.

Performance   *Criterion*   *Conditions*

Objectives

Goals identify the desired outcome performance expected to result from treatment. Frequently, however, this performance represents a large amount of change. Looking at the big picture, or "How do I get to there from here?" can be overwhelming and discouraging for the patient. Smaller steps or minigoals are needed. Objectives provide these sequential interim points to measure progress along the way to meeting the outcome goal. They increase the patient's commitment to treatment by making the outcome goal seem manageable and achievable [12,64]. For example:

Goal   Patient to work at sheltered workshop 4 hours per day in 2 months.
Objectives   1. Patient to attend to work/job in O.T. clinic for 20 minutes without
                 a break by _____.
                          (date)

2. Patient to attend to work/job in O.T. clinic for 40 minutes without a break by _____.
                                                                        (date)

In this example, dates for each objective would be determined with the patient, and they would be written along with the objectives. Objectives are sequential; one step depends on the successful completion of the step before. Not all of the steps need to be equal in size or complexity. They should, however, reflect the patient's capabilities. Your challenge is to identify objectives that are neither too small (too simple, demeaning, or boring) or too large (too overwhelming, frustrating, or demoralizing) [95]. The number of objectives for each goal depends on both the complexity of the goal and the needs of the patient. As shown in the previous example, not all objectives need to be specified at the beginning of treatment, as you may need to use your patient's progress to determine how large the steps should be and the amount of time the patient needs to accomplish them. Nevertheless, at least the first objective should be identified at the time the treatment plan is written so that the direction in which you are headed is clear. By using patient input, constantly monitoring the patient's reactions, and remaining flexible, you can adjust the objectives to meet the patient's changing needs.

Objectives follow the same rules of specificity as goals [12]. They include a performance, a criterion, and conditions. The performance is the major part of the objective and describes what your patient will be doing that indicates the goal is met. Criterion includes the qualitative parameters including the dates by when the objective will be completed. The conditions indicate the specific circumstances in which the objective will apply. Very often, the conditions replicate those of the goal. If they are clearly stated in the goal, the conditions do not need to be restated in each objective. For example:

Goal   Patient tries four new leisure interests involving other people in the next month.

Objective   1. By _____, patient _____ with _____.
               (date)   (activity)   (name of person)
            (Other objectives to be specified based on the patient's reaction to this objective.)

In this example, input from the patient is used to determine the activity, the date, and the person with whom he will do it. Based on the patient's reactions and progress, the remaining objectives could include several people, have two activities taking place in the same week, and so forth.

Objectives are not sacred, inviolate entities just because they have been committed to paper. They represent a map to guide the treatment toward the outcome goal; they should be revised and adjusted as needed.

Your Turn

Copy the goals you wrote for the last exercise in the following spaces and identify at least two possible objectives for each goal. Try to vary the number of objectives for each goal so you can practice your task analysis skills. Finally, double check to make sure the objectives contain specific performances (that is, not fuzzies), a criterion, and conditions. As with the last exercise, you have to speculate on some of the details to write a specific objective. The purpose of this exercise is to learn the process of writing objectives; accuracy of content becomes critical when you apply this process to an actual patient.

Goal 1:

    Objective:

    Objective:

    Objective:

    Objective:

Goal 2:

    Objective:

    Objective:

    Objective:

    Objective:

Goal 3:

    Objective:

    Objective:

    Objective:

    Objective:

Issues Affecting the Setting of Outcome Goals

Making Them Realistic

As mentioned earlier, the terminology of goal writing can be confusing. What is a long-term objective to some persons is a short-term goal to others. So far, you have learned that a goal represents the outcome performance, and the objectives represent the small, sequential steps needed to reach the goal. Some regulatory agencies require that you write long-term and short-term goals; however, *long* and *short* are not rigidly defined entities. Rather, they represent a quantity of time that is relative to the length of time you have to treat the patient. For instance, a long-term goal in a community treatment center might take 6 months to achieve, whereas a long-term goal on an acute inpatient unit might be reached in 3 weeks. It is obvious that not all long-term goals are equal in complexity. Long-term goals, then, are written for the outcome performance you can reasonably expect to accomplish with your patient in the time you have available. If you have only 3 weeks, then the long-term goal will be relatively simple, such as *patient will plan and prepare one meal for self without assistance before discharge.* If you had more time to work with the patient, you could choose a more complex outcome performance, such as *patient will plan, shop, and prepare two meals per day for self without assistance by (date).* So, the complexity of long-term goals is relative to the amount of time you have to work with the patient. For our purposes, short-term goals are considered equivalent to objectives. They are the intermediate, sequential steps needed to reach the long-term goals. For example:

Goal Patient will plan and prepare one meal for self without assistance before discharge.

Objectives (Short-term goals)
1. Patient will select menu for meal and make a shopping list with therapist assistance by _____ .
   (date)
2. Patient will prepare meal with therapist assistance on _____ .
   (date)
3. Patient will plan and prepare lunch for himself without therapist assistance on _____ .
   (date)

or

Goal Patient will plan, shop, and prepare two meals per day for self without assistance by _____ .
   (date)

Objectives (Short-term (goals)
1. Patient will plan breakfast for self for one week with therapist assistance by _____ .
   (date)
2. Patient will shop and prepare breakfast for one week with therapist assistance by _____ .
   (date)
3. Patient will plan, shop, and prepare breakfast for one week without therapist assistance by _____ .
   (date)
4. Patient will plan the evening meal for one week with therapist assistance by _____ .
   (date)
5. Patient will shop and prepare evening meal for one week with assistance by _____ .
   (date)

These examples represent the size of the steps needed for a particular patient. Your patient might be able to plan, shop, and prepare all in one step. Conversely, he might need to take even smaller steps. As stated earlier, goals and objectives need to be tailored to each patient's needs to be both meaningful and realistic.

Your Turn
Review the goals and objectives you have written so far, and estimate the length of time required to complete them. Since the objectives represent intermediate steps, they should be completed in the amount of time allotted to the goal. Fill in the chart below:

Goal   *Time needed*

1. _____   _____
2. _____   _____
3. _____   _____

Can any of your goals be completed in 2 or 3 weeks? If your goals take longer than that, they would be appropriate for day-treatment, outpatient, or community-based O.T. programs. Shorter time frames are appropriate for inpatient treatment programs. If none of your goals can be accomplished in 2 or 3 weeks, rewrite them to reflect this short time frame.

Goal   *Time needed*

1. _____   _____

2. _____   _____

3. _____   _____

Patient's Role

Although this topic is addressed last, it is probably the most important. You need extensive input from your patient when writing outcome goals and objectives to be successful in reaching those goals. Your treatment cannot be successful unless you identify goals, performances, criteria, conditions, and objectives that are acceptable to and endorsed by your patient. Many studies of patient involvement in goal setting convincingly suggest that involvement increases the patient's motivation, commitment to treatment, and the ultimate success of the treatment [13,77,98,102]. In a study of 82 day-treatment patients, Falloon and Talbot found that psychosocial rehabilitation efforts were most effective when the goals were primarily determined by the consumers of the mental health program. "Effectiveness of the program appeared to depend less on the excellence of the therapy than on the involvement of the patient in planning his or her goals and subsequent treatment plan" [30, p. 283].

Involving the patient in the goal-setting process implies that he is able to cooperate. If unstable or intrusive symptoms prevent the patient from participating, then the setting of outcome goals may either be delayed or modified in a manner that enables him to participate [30,102].

Setting goals (or stating *what should be*) necessitates making a value judgment about your patient; therefore, he should be involved in the process. Patient involvement in the goal-setting process enhances the patient's perception of control and thus ultimately improves both the therapeutic relationship and the treatment outcome [98]. The importance of enhanced patient control is discussed further in the section on "Treatment Implementation" (p. 148).

Your Turn

It is time to take stock of your assumptions and opinions. There is no right or wrong answer to the following questions. Answer them with your current knowledge and the understanding that your answers may change as you gain more clinical experience.

1. Do you think it is important for the patient to participate in setting the treatment goals? State your reasons.

2. To what extent should the patient be involved? (Be specific)

3. Is there any time that the patient should definitely not be involved?

4. What if the patient refuses to participate in setting treatment goals?

5. Do you believe that people can completely recover from psychiatric disorders?

Share these thoughts with a colleague or fellow student. The diversity of opinion should make for a lively and thought-provoking discussion.

Service Goals

Service goals, sometimes referred to as process goals, are written to reflect tasks for the therapist to do, not outcome behaviors expected of the patient. There was a time in the history of psychiatry when all treatment goals were written as service goals, or tasks for the professionals. Outcome goals, however, became popular in the 1960s with the increased specificity of behavioral treatment approaches. Instead of aiming for global system changes, as many service goals did, outcome goals were designed to identify specific symptoms targeted for change. Identifying these changes in the patient's performance after treatment provided both a measurable end goal and a direction for the treatment process itself. Thus, specificity in the writing of goals became desirable, and, for the most part, service goals have not been widely used in the past decade.

Allen, in her recent work on cognitive disabilities, reintroduced the concept of service goals as a viable procedure in O.T. [3]. She contends that, to date, occupational therapists have not proved their ability to meet the outcome goals they have been writing. Writing goals that cannot be substantiated damages O.T.'s credibility as a profession. "Occupational therapy was founded during a period of history when no one questioned a profession's ability to fulfill its objectives, but the times have changed. Objectives must be fulfilled, and they must be cost-effective [3, p. 27]. She suggests that environmental compensation and treatment goals are realistic for cognitively disabled patients in acute inpatient treatment programs. Because the cognitive disabilities frame of reference focuses on the therapist's task intervention, service goals make sense. They provide a guide for the therapist's interventions, but do not focus on changing the patient. Successful outcome thus would be measured by the number of goals that the *therapist* completed, rather than the amount of change that the *patient* made. Suggested service goals for this frame of reference are determined by the patient's cognitive level and psychiatric disorder. Suggested goals include [3, p. 222]:

Levels 1 and 2	Assess self-care tasks on ward.
Level 3	Assist with completion of problem-free tasks.
Level 4	Provide short-term tasks and assist with problem solving to monitor functional abilities and the disease process.
Level 5	Provide novel tasks and assist with problem solving to monitor functional abilities and the disease process.
Level 6	Provide desirable tasks and assist with observations of symptom reduction to monitor the disease process.

As with outcome goals, service goals must be measurable. Since the function of goals, in general, is to provide a guide for treatment, service goals can be measured if they clearly contain a therapist task, and not a disguised patient behavior. For instance, it is difficult to measure whether *provide opportunities for patient to express unconscious needs* has been accomplished. Successful completion of this goal implies that the patient will express unconscious needs, and that is neither the stated focus of the goal nor a measurable performance. (It does not pass the "Hey, Dad!" test.) On the other hand, *functional observations for clarification of symptoms* can be determined easily by reading the therapist's progress notes. The therapist has either done it or not, and the accomplishment of the goal does not rely on the patient making a change in his performance.

In summary, outcome goals state a desired change in some aspect(s) of the patient's functioning, and service goals represent a guide for the therapist's intervention. Both are used appropriately in the contexts given.

Your Turn

Writing measurable service goals can be tricky. Review the following list and check those goals that are not measurable. Remember, service goals should identify tasks for the therapist and should not include or imply a patient performance.

_____ 1. Provide opportunities for the patient to become aware of both his assets and his limitations
_____ 2. Provide support
_____ 3. Functional observations for titration of medicine
_____ 4. Improve the patient's interpersonal skills
_____ 5. Offer experiences for the patient to experience a sense of accomplishment
_____ 6. Monitor patient's cognitive level through his task performance
_____ 7. Evaluate patient's potential for grave disability
_____ 8. Improve the patient's self-esteem

Do you think you have it? Write an outcome goal(s), using the cognitive disabilities frame of reference, for the following problem.

Problem	Indicator	Goal
Attention span is limited to the immediate goal	Unable to maintain interest in the activity beyond one or two sessions	
	Measures time by personal needs, such as time for lunch, medications, or cigarettes	

Summary

In this section you were introduced to two types of goals: outcome and service. You learned how to relate the content of outcome goals to the patient's problems and indicators, and you learned that, in order to be specific and measurable, outcome goals should include a performance, criterion, and condition. You were introduced to objectives and also to factors that affect the setting of outcome goals. Finally, you learned how to write measurable service goals. The next section addresses the final aspect of treatment planning: selecting the methods you will use to achieve the goals.

Methods

Presently the tactful Mole slipped away and returned with a pencil and a few half-sheets of paper, which he placed on the table at his friend's elbow. "It's quite a long time since you did any poetry," he remarked. "You might have a try at it this evensong, instead of—well, brooding over things so much. I've an idea that you'll feel a lot better when you've got something jotted down."

. . . It was a joy to the Mole to know that the cure had at least begun.

Kenneth Grahame
The Wind in The Willows

Now that you have identified the goals and objectives and know what you want to try to achieve, you are ready for the final step of treatment planning: selecting the methods, or the means of accomplishing those goals. Methods includes both what you use (the activity) and how it is used (structure, teaching methods, and format).

Selecting the Activity

Background Issues

Using purposeful activities to influence a patient's health was one of the underlying tenets of the founders of the profession. Early pioneers of O.T. believed that the health of individuals could be influenced by ". . . the use of muscles and mind together in games, exercises, handicraft, and work" [47, p. 3]. The belief in the healing power of activities has, in part, defined O.T. as a profession over the years [112]. Purposeful activity is believed to prevent and remediate dysfunction and to facilitate adaptation. Nevertheless, the explosion of neuroscience literature and changes in the health-care delivery arena are challenging that treasured belief in both physical dysfunction and psychiatric practice [2,3,40,71,113]. The American Occupational Therapy Association (AOTA) position paper on purposeful activities sparked a recent debate over the usefulness of activities in the treatment of physical dysfunction [4,44,71]. It is beyond the scope of this book to discuss the use of activities in the treatment of physical dysfunction; however, a review of the relevant issues is highly recommended before you begin your fieldwork in that area. Some of the beliefs about the use of activities in psychiatric O.T. will be summarized, because they directly influence your choice of activities to meet treatment goals and objectives.

Various beliefs and assumptions about O.T.'s use of activities appear in the literature [8,22,32,49,56,70,71,80,92,93,95,113,116]. Because these beliefs are familiar and well represented in the literature, only those being re-examined are summarized below.

1. Purposeful activities can be used to restore or develop the patient's functional status by teaching him new skills or helping him relearn old ones. Active involvement in an activity provides the opportunity to learn skills by actually doing them and receiving immediate feedback from both the therapist and the nonhuman environment.
2. Purposeful activities can be used to facilitate development by structuring the treatment environment to elicit an adaptive response. Many behaviors are acquired in a developmental and age-specific sequence; thus, the treatment environment can be designed to facilitate integrated acquisition of the behavior.
3. Purposeful activities can be used to promote the patient's sense of competence and mastery through successful experiences. The just-right challenge places demands that are just above the patient's functional level. Through action with feedback, the patient becomes aware of his potential and his limits and gains a sense of competence and self-worth.

These beliefs, among others, are fundamental to the functional performance, sensory integration, and model of human occupation frames of reference. The cognitive disabilities frame of reference represents a major conceptual shift from the others in many respects. One notable difference is that the activity or task is regarded as the focus of O.T. intervention. Rather than attempting to try to change the patient, the task is changed to facilitate his maximal performance. Consequently, using activities as treatment methods is viewed differently in this frame of reference. These differences are summarized in the following sections; however a comprehensive review of Allen's recent text on cognitive disabilities [3] is needed for a thorough understanding of the issues.

Issue 1. Purposeful activities are used to teach skills. Allen argues that psychiatric illness frequently causes residual cognitive disabilities that make new learning possible for only some patients (cognitive levels 5 and 6); thus, trying to teach skills to these patients (cognitive levels 1 through 4) will be ineffective and frustrating for both you and the patient. Reviewing basic skills already known (e.g., self-care topics, using community resources, crafts, basic grooming) for these cognitively disabled patients is suggested as a more realistic and achievable objective.

Issue 2. Purposeful activities are used to stimulate acquisition of behavior in a developmental sequence. The developmental perspective may be the most useful in distinguishing the severity of the cognitive disability and to determine if it is getting better or worse. Nevertheless, applying the developmental concept to treatment objectives, especially with acute conditions, is regarded as basically misleading. Because people with acute cognitive disabilities can be expected to have a degree of spontaneous remission to premorbid levels of functioning, with or without O.T., the improvement we see may be caused by many factors, not just O.T. [3]. Statements suggesting that O.T. is responsible for the improvement (implied by treatment objectives such as *to improve* or *to increase*) are, at the moment, inaccurate and unsubstantiated claims.

Issue 3. Purposeful activity can increase the patient's sense of competency through providing the just-right challenge. Although it is sometimes possible to encourage the patient to function at a higher cognitive level, this can be frustrating for both the patient and the therapist. Especially in acute conditions, when improvement can be expected, Allen questions the rationale for forcing higher levels of functioning and suggests, rather, that the therapist make the waiting as pleasant as possible [3]. Successful task performance accompanied by a pleasant task experience is believed to provide an effective outcome of O.T. services [3, p. 187]. Pleasant task experiences and successful task performance are sought through reduction of the novelty required to do the task, not presenting an activity above the patient's functional level. Activities that expose the patient to his limitations may create catastrophic reactions (blame, anger, rage, fear, or flight) and should be avoided.

Although using purposeful activity to facilitate change may have ". . . stood the test of time" [70, p. 31], current changes in the knowledge base and demands of practice are forcing occupational therapists to reexamine some cherished beliefs. "The advances in the neurosciences are wreaking havoc on occupational therapists' view of activity. We thought that doing an activity would prevent illness or restore health. That now appears to be a naive oversimplification. As a cherished idea it has been woven through the entire fabric of our thought, and the readjustments required are major" [3, p. 27].

The previous discussion illustrates divergent views surrounding the purpose of using activities; yet all O.T. frames of reference are united in their endorsement of activity as the major treatment modality.

Selection Guidelines

Selection of activities for your patient begins with a look at the range of activities available to O.T. [96]. Unfortunately, at present the term *activity* is often interpreted to mean solely crafts. This was not always the case. The earliest definition of O.T. included the use of "any activity, mental or physical." Over the years, O.T. has lost or given away to other professions the use of play; self-expression through art, music, and dance; prevocational activities; and some activities involving daily living skills [113]. Recent efforts have been made to reacquaint occupational therapists with these areas, and the substitution of the term *occupation* for *activity* is suggested by some to reacknowledge our broader-than-craft emphasis [113]. Theoretically, therapists can use anything that is legal and that the patient wants to do [3]; yet an activity range that broad may not be feasible. There are thus both theoretic and practical constraints.

As you have learned, each frame of reference provides guidelines for the selection and use of appropriate activities. Gross motor activities designed to provide vestibular input in the sensory integration frame of reference would not be used in the same way in the cognitive disabilities frame of reference. Values clarification exercises, used in the model of human occupation and functional performance frames of reference, would not be used in the sensory integration frame of reference. Because you used a frame of reference to guide the evaluation and treatment planning process, you have identified problems and written goals that are appropriate to that frame of reference. Activity selection follows the same principles.

Most practical constraints result from limited availability of resources. The O.T. department may not have access to, or be able to purchase, major equipment such as a computer, kitchen, woodworking machines, or kiln. You may not have enough patients or time to use some types of treatment methods, such as a variety of groups, sensory integration activities, or work jobs. In addition, it may be neither cost-effective nor efficient for you to provide some types of services such as recreation or community trips. Limited resources can be a source of inspiration. Many O.T. programs ingeniously use donated supplies and equipment, volunteers or student helpers, community resources, and shared resources with other O.T. departments. The need for new equipment and expanded supplies can be justified, although this is frequently a long-term solution. Selection of activities thus requires both an understanding of the theoretic rationale for their use and the creativity to live within or overcome the practical constraints.

Although the frames of reference differ in many respects, all endorse the principle that the activity selected should be meaningful to the patient. "The meaning of the activity, its choice, and satisfaction in it are determined by the individual patient's needs, interests, and motivations. They should *not* be determined by the occupational therapists' view of meaning" [116, p. 27]. Who actually selects the activity, the therapist or the patient, differs with the frame of reference. Generally, however, some parameters are provided by the therapist, and some choices are provided for the patient within these guidelines. Specific guidance and rationales for activity selection are provided by each frame of reference.

The age- and gender-appropriateness of the activity affect both its perceived meaningfulness and the patient's motivation to participate. For instance, some men may find sewing or cooking demeaning, whereas others may not. Some women may find woodworking unfeminine, whereas others may not. Some people over 30 may regard making collages on the same level as cutting out paper dolls. Obviously, if your patient is uncomfortable or even offended by the activity selected, he is not going to benefit from it. Activity selection becomes the most problematic when the patient's functional abilities are more impaired than his verbal abilities. Such patients are often unaware of this discrepancy and regard the activities they are able to accomplish successfully in O.T. as too simple or too childish. Increasing the complexity of the task, however, often results in failure and frustration. This complex situation must be handled sensitively. You can thoroughly check the patient's interests, provide choices, and monitor his response to the activity. You can structure whatever activity he chooses so that he can succeed at it. Whether or not you point out this discrepancy in functioning to the patient depends on your frame of reference and the philosophy of the treatment program within which you are working. Most of all, do not become personally offended when your patient tells you that the activity is stupid or childish. It might be . . . for him. Use this feedback to help select an activity that is more suitable for him. Arguing about the intended purpose of the activity or its inherent value is useless. No activity is useful unless the patient finds it meaningful.

Finally, the activity selected must match the problem and the goal and call upon the patient's strengths.

Example 1: Functional Performance
Problem   Feels inferior to peers. Has not initiated contact with peers in past 6 months.

Goal   Attend movie with peers two times in the next month.

Methods   *Activities*—assertiveness or social-skills activities, such as developing friendships, introducing self, and expressing self to others.

In this example, it is presumed that you know (from your assessment) that the reason the patient has not initiated contact with peers is that he feels inadequate about his communication skills. The purpose of the treatment is to teach communication skills and thus increase his confidence with his peers. The activities selected address this goal directly. Although it could be argued that other activities, such as gross motor activities or successful experiences at crafts or cooking, could help the patient feel better about himself, they do not address the goal directly and therefore are not appropriate. As you recall from the problem list (Table 2-2) this patient's strengths include valuing friendships and having interests that can provide contact with peers. If these strengths are used in the goals and methods, they can help motivate the patient to participate.

Example 2: Sensory Integration
Problem   Impaired balance. Lost balance on Romberg in 4/4 trials. Unable to hold sharpened Romberg for 10 seconds.

Goal   Able to perform Romberg with no difficulty in 4/4 trials and to hold sharpened Romberg for 30 seconds.

Methods   *Activities*—gross motor activities that require shifting balance and standing on one leg, such as throwing and catching ball, skipping, and simple exercises.

In this example, the purpose of the treatment is to help the patient improve his balance by participating in different activities that require using balance. It is presumed that you have already assessed his interests and selected those possible to accomplish at your treatment facility before selecting those stated above. Other activities such as basketball, balance board, or dancing may meet the goal, but be discarded because of lack of interest or resources. Recall from your assessment (Table 2-3) that this patient has adequate muscle strength and sitting balance. You know that strengthening exercises are not needed, and you can start with active, standing-balance activities.

Example 3: Model of Human Occupation

Problem	Current role performance imbalance: discrepancy between valued roles and actual performance.
Goal	Participate in two activities of valued role (hobbyist) in the next 2 weeks.
Methods	*Activities*—quilting and planting terrariums.

In this example, the purpose of the treatment is to help the patient start doing those activities she values, but for some reason does not currently do. It is presumed that you thoroughly checked the patient's interests before deciding on these two activities. It could be argued that self-awareness or value-clarification activities would help the patient understand more about herself, however, they do not carry out the intent of the treatment—to mobilize the patient to participate—and are not appropriate for this goal. As you recall from your assessment (Table 2-4) this patient's strengths include valuing a variety of roles and a history of successful role performance, thus providing further indication for facilitating participation rather than values clarification.

Example 4: Cognitive Disabilities

Problem	Does not invent new motor actions. Does not correct errors with demonstrated solutions. Unable to retain two-step directions.
Goal	Provide short-term tasks and assist with patient problem solving to monitor functional ability and symptoms.
Methods	*Activities*—patient choice of basic skills review, such as self-care topics or using community resources, and intellectual skills and crafts, such as making a wooden box, decoupage, or leather key cases.

In this example, the purpose of the treatment is to use the activity both for continued assessment and for palliative and supportive treatment. The therapist clearly provides help with problem solving to minimize the patient's frustration resulting from trying an activity he is unable to do. Your assessment (Table 2-5) indicated that one of this patient's strengths was that his actions were goal directed; thus, short-term, meaningful activities are indicated. It might be argued that other activities to learn problem solving, such as learning the steps or behavioral rehearsal, would be appropriate. This combination of problems, goals, and methods is based on the cognitive deficiencies frame of reference, which strives to facilitate the patient's best performance by making the task possible for him to do rather than attempting to change the patient in some way. Activities that try to teach the patient how to solve problems are thus not appropriate for this frame of reference.

Many factors are involved in selecting activities to achieve your treatment goals and objectives (see Fig. 3-1). At first, this selection process may seem laborious, but, like all other skills, it becomes easier as you gain experience. Before long, it will be second nature to run quickly through this list in your head as you select activities!

Your Turn

In the last section, you wrote at least three outcome goals and one service goal. Select at least three activities for each of these goals. Review Tables 2-2 through 2-5 for additional information about the patient's problems and strengths. Although you will not know what the patient's interests are or the resource constraints of your facility, this exercise will give you practice in generating activity ideas.

Fig. 3-1. A guide for the
selection of activities.

_____ Name of Ax

Yes   No

——   ——   Is the activity appropriately used with the frame of reference employed
             so far in the assessment and treatment planning process? Rationale:

——   ——   Does the treatment facility have the resources to use this activity? Ration-
             ale:

——   ——   If not, can the resources be found elsewhere to enable use of the activity
             with this patient? Rationale:

——   ——   Is the activity meaningful to the patient? Rationale:

——   ——   Is the activity appropriate for the patient's age and gender? Rationale:

——   ——   Does the activity match the problem and the goal? Rationale:

——   ——   Does the activity capitalize on the patient's strengths? Rationale:

Goal   *Activity*

Once you have selected the activities for each goal, use the checklist in Fig. 3-1 to determine if they are appropriate. You should be able to justify your selection on each
of the points listed.

Using the Activity

Selecting the activity is only half of the task; using it effectively is the other half.
Once selected, the activity must be individualized to meet each patient's needs and
goals. Individualizing the activity requires determining the best structure, teaching
methods, and format for each patient.

Selecting the Structure

Structuring an activity means to analyze its component processes, materials, and
tools and to sequence these into steps based on a system of logic [80,92]. Activity
analysis and synthesis have been identified as legitimate tools of O.T. and are used
by all frames of reference [80]. As noted in the section on "Role of Theory" (p. 112),
each frame of reference postulates the nature of O.T. intervention and the resulting
positive change in the patient. Activities are thus analyzed to determine if they fit
these postulates and synthesized to determine how they can be used within that
theoretic framework. For example, activities in the functional performance frame

of reference would be analyzed for their psychologic, social, motor, sensory integrative, and cognitive components, as well as age and cultural relevance [33], whereas the sensory integration frame of reference would analyze activities for their vestibular, proprioceptive, and tactile qualities [43]. Each frame of reference thus proposes analysis of different components of activities. Thorough analysis is the first step. The second step is synthesis or presenting the activity to your patient in an organized, sequenced manner that will achieve the treatment goals. Reed identifies several universal approaches to structuring tasks [92].

1. *Normal developmental sequencing.* Activity steps are sequenced according to the way they normally occur in childhood and adult development (e.g., balance is achieved before walking; dependence is expected before independence).
2. *Normal activity sequencing.* Activity steps are sequenced according to the manner in which the activity normally occurs (e.g., dishes are washed after eating; make-up is put on after shower).
3. *Adapted/structured sequencing.* Activity steps are adapted to enable more independent completion (e.g., complex steps are broken down into smaller units; novelty is reduced; steps are omitted by using kits or mixes). Allen's extensive activity analysis for persons with cognitive disabilities provides much practical and useful information for adapting/structuring activities [1,3].

How do you decide which of these structures to use? Factors that affect selection include the goal of treatment, the frame of reference used, the patient, and the activity itself. The examples below illustrate structure selection for the activities chosen in the last section.

Example 1: Functional Performance

Problem   Feels inferior to peers. Has not initiated contact with peers in past 6 months.

Goal   Attend movie with peers two times in the next month.

Methods   *Activities*—assertiveness or social skills activities, such as developing friendships, introducing self, and expressing self to others.
Structure—normal activity sequencing.

Because communication happens in a sequential manner (introduce self, find topics of mutual interest to discuss, listen, demonstrate nonverbal and verbal interest, express feelings, give and receive feedback) structuring the social skills activities used for treatment to simulate the normal course of communication is the best choice. Once the structure is decided, you would plan how many sessions you would need to teach these skills and which topics would be included in each session. A possible sequence is suggested below:

Session 1: Meeting new people
Session 2: Listening skills
Session 3: Expressing yourself
Session 4: Giving and receiving feedback

Example 2: Sensory Integration

Problem   Impaired balance. Lost balance on Romberg in 4/4 trials. Unable to hold sharpened Romberg for 10 seconds.

Goal   Able to perform Romberg with no difficulty in 4/4 trials and to hold sharpened Romberg for 30 seconds.

Methods   *Activities*—gross motor activities that require shifting balance and standing on one leg, such as throwing and catching ball, skipping, and simple exercises.
Structure—normal developmental sequencing.

Balance is normally acquired in a developmental sequence. You learn to sit up, stand up, balance on one foot, keep your balance when jostled, balance while moving, and balance when your attention is distracted by another activity. Because one of the principles of the sensory integration frame of reference is to provide sensory input in a developmentally appropriate sequence, simulating normal development is the best choice of activity structure. Next, sequence the activities you plan to do with the patient to fit the structure. A beginning sequence is described below:

Shift balance from foot to foot.
Shift balance from foot to foot with attention distracted.
Stand on one leg.
Stand on one leg with attention distracted.

Example 3: Model of Human Occupation
Problem   Current role performance imbalance: discrepancy between valued roles and actual performance.
Goal   Participate in two activities of valued role (hobbyist) in the next 2 weeks.
Methods   *Activities*—quilting and planting terrariums.
Structure—adapted/structured sequencing.

Based on the results of your assessment, you predict that this patient should have no difficulty completing either of these two activities if they are broken down in step-by-step directions. Adapted/structured sequencing is the best choice for structuring these activities for this patient. Most craft instructions are written in a step-by-step manner. If the patient is able to read and follow directions, no further adapting of the activity is necessary.

Example 4: Cognitive Disabilities
Problem   Does not invent new motor actions. Does not correct errors with demonstrated solutions. Unable to retain two-step directions.
Goal   Provide short-term tasks and assist with patient problem solving to monitor functional ability and symptoms.
Methods   *Activities*—patient choice of basic skills review, such as self-care topics or using community resources, and intellectual skills and crafts, such as making a wooden box, decoupage, or leather key cases.
Structure—adapted/structures sequencing.

Based on the results of your assessment, this patient is functioning at cognitive level 4. These activities would be structured accordingly to facilitate the patient's maximal functioning. Some ways to structure an activity for a level 4 patient are suggested below [3]:

An exact sample must be available.
The activity must be able to be completed in one session.
Pieces must be precut and holes punched.

Directions must be demonstrated as well as verbal.
Directions must be given one step at a time.

Your Turn
Select a structure for each of the activities chosen in the last section. Write a justification for that structure in the spaces provided.

Activity   *Structure*

Rationale:

Rationale:

Rationale:

Rationale:

Selecting Teaching Methods
Although occupational therapists have not always welcomed the title of teacher (especially craft teacher), the teaching-learning process has been identified as another of O.T.'s legitimate tools [80]. Reed suggests that once the activity is selected and the structure determined, the teaching method, or the way the activity is presented to the patient, can be identified [92]. Your experience of getting an education has given you an intimate familiarity with didactic teaching methods such as lectures, discussions, homework assignments, and audiovisual (AV) aids. Since many occupational therapists believe in learning by doing, experiential learning methods are also applicable. Several of these are described below:

1. *Demonstration and performance.* The desired behavior (performance) is demonstrated by the therapist and copied by the patient [92]. This method is particularly useful when the behavior to be learned is either a novel physical action (e.g., lifting a parachute, operating power woodworking equipment, or breaking an egg), or complex and difficult for the patient to complete on his own. In both instances, demonstrated behaviors reduce the novelty of the task by using imitation of a role model. Then asking the patient to perform the behavior, rather than just watching you, helps him learn by actually doing it and receiving feedback from you about his performance. Generalization of the newly learned behavior is often problematic and must be specifically addressed when using this method.
2. *Explore and discover.* Various activities are arranged, and the patient is allowed to explore any or all of them to discover what happens. Used with children and endorsed as one method in the model of human occupation, it is useful to encourage interest and investment in the activity. Because this method is basically self-directed, the therapist has little control over the amount, type, or quality of the patient's performance [92].

3. *Role play.* Participants assume a given perspective or set of behaviors and act them out in a fantasy or pretend situation. Role play is particularly useful to practice or test new skills, such as assertiveness, communication, or interviewing. Because it also enhances the participants' awareness of the feelings, attitudes, and behaviors of others, role play can be used to promote an attitude change. It can also be quite threatening to the participants and must be used discriminately and with caution [110].

4. *Problem solving.* The therapist teaches the patient to examine the problem situation, define the problem, brainstorm possible alternatives, weigh each alternative, select one, try it out, and evaluate the results. Problem solving is particularly useful for dealing with life situations such as finding a job or locating an apartment in a new city. Once the process is learned, it can be generalized to many situations. Nevertheless, learning the process can be time-consuming, and several trial and error attempts are to be expected before the skill is learned [92].

5. *Written tasks.* Using a diary or log book to document what the patient is learning helps to sustain his attention and strengthen his memory. A log can also serve as a basis for self-evaluation over time and a record of the patient's progress. Paper-and-pencil tasks provide low-risk involvement when direct interpersonal interaction might be too threatening [110]. Written tasks also provide a personalized, private means of self-exploration. The patient can write his thoughts and feelings and continue to work with the topic after the O.T. session. Written tasks are more effective if feedback from the therapist and other patients is included. One disadvantage to written tasks is that the therapist may have difficulty assessing the patient's current status and reactions to the activity if he is unwilling to share what he wrote with the therapist.

6. *Projects and field trips.* Projects and field trips offer an opportunity for the patient to integrate his newly learned skills in a context outside the O.T. clinic [110]. Banking can be done at the patient's bank, information on community resources gathered from local agencies, grocery shopping done at the supermarket. Projects and field trips aid in generalization of the skill being learned, but require significantly more time, effort, and money.

7. *Audiovisual aids.* Audiovisual aids such as movies, filmstrips, photographs, overhead projections, graphs, or blackboard diagrams can be used effectively to clarify and illustrate points, stimulate discussion, or demonstrate something that cannot be recreated in the O.T. clinic. Audiovisual presentations are enhanced by discussion and feedback to personalize what has been seen for each patient [110]. Although AV can be very effective, it is often difficult to obtain materials that relate directly to your patient population. Producing your own is both costly and time-consuming.

8. *Body movement.* Body movement can be used for a variety of purposes from relaxation to developing personal awareness. Movement has the major advantage of providing access to some issues that verbal methods do not, such as how a relaxed body actually feels. Movement, however, is often threatening and must be used with discrimination [110].

Lecturing, explaining, and other forms of didactic instruction were purposely omitted from this list. Certainly some verbal exchange occurs with these other methods, but you can be more creative in your selection of experiential learning methods if you limit the didactic exchanges to those inherent in the other methods.

The use of experiential teaching methods is not without problems, the most notable of which is lack of generalization of the learning to the patient's life outside the treatment setting. In many instances, you set up treatment situations that are similar to analogue observations (see Chap. 2 for review); thus generalization is not guaranteed. Techniques to help increase generalization have been suggested [39,110] and should be incorporated into treatment.

Which method(s) should you use? In part, the method is determined by the type of activity chosen, the skill being learned, the resources available, and the patient's needs and preferences. In other words, the choice must be individualized for each patient. You can also select more than one teaching method for each activity. Because few clinical studies have examined which methods are effective with which problems/goals/activities, this decision is based primarily on clinical judgment. Studying which methods are most effective for a specific problem holds promise for exciting and badly needed clinical research. Teaching methods have been selected for the previously used examples.

Example 1: Functional Performance

Problem   Feels inferior to peers. Has not initiated contact with peers in past 6 months.

Goal   Attend movie with peers two times in the next month.

Methods   *Activities*—assertiveness or social skills activities, such as developing friendships, introducing self, and expressing self to others.

         Structure—normal activity sequencing.

         Teaching methods—demonstration and performance, role play, written tasks.

In this example, social skills could be taught using the methods listed above. Some content (e.g., nonverbal expressiveness, displaying verbal interest, giving feedback) might be best taught with demonstration and performance. The patient could observe the therapist role-model the novel behavior and then practice it. Role play would be an effective way to practice newly learned skills in anticipated difficult situations. For example, if the patient expected that asking a peer to the movies would be difficult, the situation could be role-played with the therapist providing a variety of responses to help the patient decide what he would say in the actual situation. Written tasks could be used to evaluate the patient's social skills further as well as to assess his progress. They could also be used as homework assignments to help integrate the information learned in the O.T. session.

Example 2: Sensory Integration

Problem   Impaired balance. Lost balance on Romberg in 4/4 trials. Unable to hold sharpened Romberg for 10 seconds.

Goal   Able to perform Romberg with no difficulty in 4/4 trials and to hold sharpened Romberg for 30 seconds.

Methods   *Activities*—gross motor activities that require shifting balance and standing on one leg, such as throwing and catching ball, skipping, and simple exercises.

         Structure—normal developmental sequencing.

         Teaching method—body movement.

Body movement is the only logical teaching method that would facilitate working on the patient's balance.

Example 3: Model of Human Occupation

Problem   Current role performance imbalance: discrepancy between valued roles and actual performance.

Goal   Participate in two activities of valued role (hobbyist) in the next 2
              weeks.

Methods   *Activities*—quilting and planting terrariums.
              Structure—adapted/structured sequencing.
              Teaching methods—explore and discover, AV aids, projects and field
              trips.

Based on your assessment, it appears that this patient does not have significant impairments in functional capacities. The explore-and-discover teaching methods may
help to stimulate this patient's interests. Materials, directions, pictures of completed work, and samples would be laid out to encourage the patient's experimen-
tation. In addition to the pictures, other AV aids might include a videotape of the
process or a book about its history. For instance, the patient could make a field trip
to the nursery to buy plants for the terrariums or to the art museum to view quilts.

Example 4: Cognitive Disabilities

Problem   Does not invent new motor actions. Does not correct errors with dem-
              onstrated solutions. Unable to retain two-step directions.

Goal   Provide short-term tasks and assist with patient problem solving to
              monitor functional ability and symptoms.

Methods   *Activities*—patient choice of basic skills review, such as self-care topics
              or using community resources, and intellectual skills and crafts,
              such as making a wooden box, decoupage, or leather key cases.
              Structure—adapted/structured sequencing.
              Teaching method—demonstration and performance.

Given the cognitive limitations of a person functioning at level 4, the demonstration and performance method is the best choice. Specific guidance for using this
method with cognitively impaired patients has been extensively provided
elsewhere [3].

Your Turn

Select teaching methods for each of the activities chosen in the last section. Certainly you may use more than one method, but more than three will become unwieldy.
Write a justification for the methods you selected in the spaces provided.

Activity   *Teaching methods*   *Rationale*

Selecting the Format

Finally, you need to decide whether the treatment should occur in a group or individual treatment format; each has its advantages and disadvantages.

1. *Group format.* Treating patients in groups has a long history in psychiatric O.T. practice. Even though patients have been treated in groups for many years, using the group process itself as an agent of change did not become popular until the late 1950s [28,92]. Treating patients in a group provides several advantages. First, groups provide a format for learning skills normally learned in group settings, such as social skills and cooperation with others [78,103]. Second, groups permit the patient to receive feedback from both the other group members and the activity experience. This feedback helps to develop his sense of competence and mastery [32]. Third, conducting treatment in groups increases the therapist's productivity, as more patients can be seen in a shorter time. Finally, groups are versatile and can be used with a variety of content areas.

   The use of groups also has several disadvantages, mostly specific to small, acute-care facilities. The rapid turnover of patients and short lengths of stay in acute treatment settings prohibit the development of the group cohesiveness necessary to use the group process fully as an agent of change. Since new patients are constantly entering, groups frequently stay at the getting-to-know-you, polite stages [17]. In addition, patients who are functioning at different levels with different needs are difficult to treat together in some types of group structure. For instance, patients who are acutely symptomatic are often easily distracted and disturbed by the noise and stimulation that normally accompany a group. Patients with higher levels of functioning find the group boring and demeaning if the content is too simple or the pace too slow. As with any activity, the patient has a negative experience when he and the group are not accurately matched. Yet, resource constraints, especially in small facilities, often prevent the provision of all the groups that would be useful in meeting each patient's needs.

2. *Individual treatment format.* Treating patients individually has several advantages. It allows concentrated effort on each of the patient's goals, thus increasing the chances that they can be met. Because the amount and type of sensory stimulation can be controlled more easily in individual sessions, acutely ill patients can be treated earlier in their hospital stay. Individual treatment allows extreme flexibility in the selection of methods and responses to the patient's changing needs. For example, changes in the patient's treatment program can be made quickly because no major O.T. program change is required and only you and the patient are involved. The major disadvantages to using individual treatment are that it is time-consuming, expensive, and it limits the number of patients that can be seen daily. In addition, individual treatment minimizes the opportunities for mutual support and problem solving that could be gained from other group members.

Neither format is "better" under all circumstances. The best solution is to incorporate the positive features and minimize the negative features of each to meet the needs of the patient population you are serving.

ACTIVITY OR VERBAL?

Through the years, occupational therapists have facilitated a potpourri of groups. Despite the preponderance of activity groups reported in the literature and the declaration of activity groups as a legitimate tool of O.T. [80], apparently verbal therapy groups are also widespread in psychiatric O.T. [28,53].

For years, occupational therapists have philosophically believed that activity groups are more effective than verbal groups in developing interpersonal skills, and studies from outside the profession provide some support for these notions. Studies of social skills training reviewed by Brady suggest that skill training in a group, involving the use of structured instruction, modeling, practice, and feedback, is an effective way to teach social skills [14,15]. Although these studies have some methodologic problems (most notable is the failure to control for differences in psychiatric diagnosis), the results suggest that social skills can be taught more effectively by having the patient learn and practice them in a group than by talking about them.

Recent studies in O.T. are also starting to provide support for the belief that activity groups are valuable in developing interpersonal skills. Because this issue is important, the following three studies are reported in some detail.

Mumford compared the effects of verbal (n = 12) and activity (n = 12) groups on the development of interpersonal skills in students enrolled in adult education programs [82]. Each group met once a week for 3-hour sessions over a 4-month period. The Fundamental Interpersonal Relations Orientation Behavior Test was used as the pretest and post-test measure of interpersonal skills. Results indicated that the students in the activity group showed significantly more improvement in interpersonal skills than those in the verbal group.

DeCarlo and Mann replicated and expanded this study by comparing the effects of activity (n = 7) and verbal (n = 6) groups on self-reported interpersonal skills in male psychiatric patients [23]. Both groups were compared with a control group (n = 6) that received normal-milieu therapy. Each experimental group met once a week for 1-hour sessions over an 8-week period. The Interpersonal Communication Inventory was used as the pretest and post-test measure of self-reported interpersonal skills. Results indicated that the interpersonal skills of the activity group increased significantly compared to those of the verbal group ($P < 0.05$), but neither group performed significantly better than the control group. This study had some methodologic limitations; however, the results suggest that activity groups may improve the self-perception of increased interpersonal skills in psychiatric patients.

Schwartzberg, Howe, and McDermott compared the efficacy of three treatment-group formats (community, open O.T., and self-expression) in facilitating social interaction among psychiatric inpatients [101]. They found differences in both the quantity and type of interaction within the groups. The open O.T. group (a parallel task group in which each patient chose and carried out an individual activity based on his goals and interests) was characterized by the greatest amount of interaction between individual patients, more task-oriented communication, and fewer non-communicating participants. More positive social-emotional comments occurred in the open O.T. group than in the other two groups. The self-expression group (a combination task- and process-oriented group designed to facilitate verbal and non-verbal expression) had fewer noncommunicating patients than the community group, more positive social-emotional comments, and more patient-to-entire-group comments than the community group. In summary, the two O.T. groups using activities were characterized by more interaction among patients of a positive social-emotional and help-giving nature.

Although the results are not definitive, these studies suggest that activity groups may be more effective in increasing interpersonal skills than verbal groups. They need to be replicated and expanded to control for differences in diagnosis and teaching methods, and also examined for the long-term persistence of change. They do offer some beginning support for the notion that something valuable is happening when activities are used in treatment. Understanding the exact nature of the benefits activity groups hold for psychiatric patients is one critical and exciting challenge facing our profession in the next decade.

GROUP CONTENT

What content has not been covered in an O.T. group? Published descriptions of O.T. groups run the alphabet from activities of daily living [9,86,89,107] to women's identification [26]. Other O.T. groups described in the literature include: poetry [91], soap operas [29], video [24,41,45], emotions identification [5], social skills training [15], stress management [81,111], money management [51], relaxation [62], vocational training [27,46,60,61,88,89], independent living skills [83], chorus, greenhouse, active sports, leisure planning, young adults, home arts, career preparation for women, reality orientation [34], basic crafts, sewing, grooming, basic skills, clay and mosaics, work evaluation, advanced crafts [3], movement [65], library skills [48], music [76], self-expression [28], and sensory integration [20,94].

Duncombe and Howe recently surveyed 200 occupational therapists of all specialities to determine their use of groups [28]. Their results indicate that activities of daily living (17%), reality-oriented discussion (15.5%), sensorimotor/sensory integration activities (13.5%), and arts and crafts groups (10.5%) are the most frequently used. No data were provided on differences between therapists working in psychiatry and other specialities, although the authors reported that activities of daily living, cooking, tasks, arts and crafts, self-expression, feeling-oriented discussion, and reality-oriented discussion were found most commonly in psychiatric hospitals. This survey adds to our knowledge that group work is prevalent in psychiatric O.T. practice (all of the psychiatric occupational therapists responding to the survey used groups) and suggests some of the most frequently used group content.

All in all, occupational therapists cover a variety of contents in a group format. This vast diversity reveals O.T.'s broad domain of concern, variety of theoretic differences, and, probably, professional entrepreneurship. (That is, the therapist who sees a need and fills it.) It also makes it difficult to describe O.T. services to the layperson. Selection of content for a group should follow the same guidelines as selection of activities for individuals. (Review Fig. 3-1.)

GROUP STRUCTURE

The way in which the group's membership and activities are organized is called the group structure. Mosey proposes a classification system of group structures that includes the following categories [80].

1. *Task-oriented groups.* Originally conceived by Fidler [32], task-oriented groups aim to increase the patient's awareness of the interaction between his thoughts and his actions while he works on a shared task with others. "The shared decision-making, working experiences available in these groups and the opportunity to explore and work through problems that interfere with satisfactory function make integrated learning possible" [32, p. 151]. Examples of task groups include cooking a meal, making a poster, putting out a newsletter, and planning and taking a community trip.

2. *Developmental groups.* Originally conceived by Mosey [78], developmental groups aim to teach interpersonal skills through providing structure to the learning process. Developmental groups are based on the concept that group interaction skills are learned in a developmental sequence occurring in specific stages. These five stages are simulated by structured group levels (parallel, project, egocentric-cooperative, cooperative, and mature). It is believed that persons progress through these stages in a sequential manner and that simulating this natural process by progressing the patient through the levels in a group setting facilitates his development of interpersonal skills. This basic structure has been expanded and refined with the addition of goals, behavioral characteristics, and size and time factors for each group level [109].

3. *Thematic groups.* Thematic groups aim to help the patient acquire the knowledge, skills, or attitudes he needs in a certain area [80]. Sensorimotor, basic living skills, leisure planning, and self-awareness are examples of thematic groups because they are limited to a specific topic. Within this thematic structure, further divisions can be made to suit the patient's needs. For instance, the group could be divided into a basic level group that needs direction, support, and active intervention from the therapist, and an advanced level group in which the therapist serves as a coordinator or resource guide.

4. *Instrumental groups.* Instrumental groups aim to meet the patient's health needs to maintain his function [80]. By structuring activities for each individual, instrumental groups can be used to meet palliative and supportive treatment goals [3]. Patients are seen in a group, but the group process is not analyzed and used as a treatment intervention. The focus of the group is on meeting individual patients' needs through successful and pleasant task performance.

Selecting the structure of the group best suited to your patient's needs follows similar principles as selecting the structure of individual activities. The following examples illustrate the selection of group format, content, and structure.

Example 1: Functional Performance

Problem Feels inferior to peers. Has not initiated contact with peers in 6 months.
Goal Attend movie with peers two times in the next month.
Methods *Activities*—assertiveness or social skills activities, such as developing friendships, introducing self, and expressing self to others.
   Structure—normal activity sequencing.
   Teaching methods—demonstration and performance, role play.
   Format—group.
    Content: social skills.
    Structure: thematic and task group.

Since social skills require interaction with other people, teaching them in a group devoted to that topic (thematic) is a good choice. In this instance, the sequence of learning activities planned for each patient would be carried out with the whole group. With some progress, the patient could also participate in a task group in which he helps to plan a community trip to the movies and takes the initiative to ask other patients to attend.

Example 2: Sensory Integration

Problem Impaired balance. Lost balance on Romberg in 4/4 trials. Unable to hold sharpened Romberg for 10 seconds.
Goal Able to perform Romberg with no difficulty in 4/4 trials and to hold sharpened Romberg for 30 seconds.
Methods *Activities*—gross motor activities that require shifting balance and standing on one leg, such as throwing and catching a ball, skipping, and simple exercises.
   Structure—normal developmental sequencing.
   Teaching method—body movement.
   Format—individual treatment.

Although it is possible in larger treatment settings to have enough patients with sensory integration treatment goals to form a thematic group, it is unlikely in a small treatment setting. This treatment would thus be carried out individually. If it were conducted in a group, the content would be sensory integration, and the structure would be thematic.

Example 3: Model of Human Occupation

Problem — Current role performance imbalance: discrepancy between valued roles and actual performance.

Goal — Participate in two activities of valued role (hobbyist) in the next two weeks.

Methods — *Activities*—quilting and planting terrariums.
Structure—adapted/structured sequencing.
Teaching methods—explore and discover, AV aids.
Format—individual/group.
    Content: crafts.
    Structure: developmental.

This example illustrates a progression from individual to group treatment. It is presumed that the person needs individual attention to begin involvement. He could progress to a parallel group, a developmental group in which each person works on a similar task in the presence of others. If all goes well, he could work his way up the group levels until he was able to work cooperatively with others on a shared task in a mixed-gender group (mature).

Example 4: Cognitive Disabilities

Problem — Does not invent new motor actions. Does not correct errors with demonstrated solutions. Unable to retain two-step directions.

Goal — Provide short-term tasks and assist with patient problem solving to monitor functional ability and symptoms.

Methods — *Activities*—patient choice of basic skills review, such as self-care topics or using community resources, and intellectual skills and crafts, such as making a wooden box, decoupage, or leather key cases.
Structure—adapted/structured sequencing.
Teaching method—demonstration and performance.
Format—individual or group.
    Content: crafts, basic skills.
    Structure: instrumental.

Cognitively impaired patients (at level 4) can be treated either in instrumental groups or in individual sessions depending on the constraints of the O.T. program.

USING GROUPS EFFECTIVELY

The information on effective group facilitation is extensive and is not repeated here. Nevertheless, because this is an important and necessary skill, the topic is discussed briefly as it affects treatment planning. After reading the previous example, you might wonder how individual goals for five or six patients can all be met in one group. Orchestrating these goals is possible, if you take several factors into consideration during the treatment-planning phase. Different group contents and structures lend themselves to fulfilling different treatment objectives. Patients thus must be matched carefully with the group that best suits their needs. For instance, most thematic groups, such as basic living skills, self-awareness, or sensory integration, are most effective with homogeneous populations with similar problems and goals. Developmental (particularly parallel) and instrumental groups can tolerate a wide variety of patient goals, as the patients work alone while in the presence of others.

Task groups can accomodate a range of patient functioning, and, if facilitated effectively, can be a good lesson in tolerance and learning to find a productive role for everyone. Crafts are the most versatile activity; they can be structured to meet each patient's individual goals in a group treatment setting. It is possible that you could have a group of several patients who each has different goals to accomplish. It behooves you to be organized and to identify, before the group starts, what you are expecting for each patient. Unless you review what you intend to accomplish during each treatment session, the days will slip by with little progress made. Do not despair! With continued experience, you will develop skill at facilitating groups and meeting the goals of different patients in a group format. After all, if there were nothing left to learn, why have fieldwork?

STARTING A NEW GROUP

What if no group exists at your treatment facility that can meet your patient's needs? If the goal needs to be treated in a group format, start a new group. Planning new groups can be facilitated by using a protocol. Protocols follow several formats. Figure 3-2 is an example.

In general, protocols contain the following items: title, purpose, justification, goals, content, structure, logistics, patient selection, and criteria for discharge from the group. The *title* is more important than you may think at first. A rose by any other name may still be a rose, but calling it a stinkweed does not encourage you to pick it up and smell it. Similarly, group titles that simply describe the purpose in nonclinical terms may help to increase the patient's interest and motivation to participate in the group. For instance, which catches your eye: Career Planning for Women or Female Vocational Readiness? The *purpose* of the group is a short description of what the group is intended to accomplish. The *justification* includes a description of why this group is important (timely, needed, and cost-effective) and how it fits within the overall context of the O.T. department and the treatment facility's mission. Careful attention to the justification can help garner administrative support for the group. The *goals* specify what each participant is expected to achieve in the group. In addition, state both the *content* and the *structure* of the group you have planned. The *logistics* include a description of the location and time of the meeting, and the length of the sessions. The maximum number of patients desired and the names of the therapists facilitating the group are also included. The final two aspects are *selection* and *discharge criteria* for patient participation in the group. Patient selection criteria identify specific characteristics that indicate which patients could benefit from the group. It serves as a guide for other staff members to refer appropriate patients to the group. Similarily, the discharge criteria identify the outcomes needed to discontinue the patient's participation in the group.

Group protocols can also be used to document the services offered; educate professionals in other disciplines about the types, goals, and purposes of the O.T. groups; and increase appropriate referrals by specifying the types of patient problems appropriate for each group [34]. In general, writing protocols for all O.T. groups, ongoing or new, is a good and useful habit to develop.

Your Turn

For each of the activities you have identified so far, choose the treatment format. If a group format is selected, identify both the group content and the group structure. If an individual format is selected, ignore the content and structure columns. Justify your choices in the spaces provided.

Fig. 3-2. A protocol for
establishing a new
therapy group.

Title:

Purpose of group:

Justification for group:

Group goals:

Group content:

Group structure:

Logistics:

  Place:

  Meeting schedule:

  Length of session:

  Number of patients:

  Group facilitators:

Selection criteria for patients:

Discharge criteria for patients:

Source: Fidler, G. S. *Design of Rehabilitation Services in Psychiatric Hospital Settings.* Laurel, MD: Ramsco, 1984.

Activity	*Format*	*Content*	*Structure*

Rationale:

Rationale:

Rationale:

Rationale:

Rationale:

Rationale:

Rationale:

Rationale:

Rationale:

Rationale:

Summary
This section has taken you step by step through the last phase of treatment planning: methods selection. You learned how to select an activity, and how to choose the structure, teaching methods, and format for using that activity effectively. The next section of this chapter addresses the actual implementation of your treatment and the assessment of the outcome.

Implementing and Evaluating Treatment

To my audience, without whom I would only be myself.

Steve Martin
Dedication to Cruel Shoes

The assessment and initial planning are completed; now you are ready to start treatment. Because you have selected the activity, structure, teaching methods, and format, you know what you are going to do in treatment with your patient. The final step is to determine how you are going to do it, and how to determine if it does any good.

Implementing Treatment

Your knowledge of psychiatric disorders and frames of reference provides guidelines for implementing the treatment you have planned. In addition, you will begin to learn the nuts and bolts of making the treatment effective during your fieldwork. Perhaps the most important key in treatment implementation is the therapeutic relationship between you and the patient. This relationship is frequently conceived of as the most important ingredient regardless of the type of therapy employed [38,63,106]. Occupational therapy shares these beliefs. Frank's classic article on the therapeutic use of self points out that "one of the tasks of the occupational therapist is to use himself to help the patient develop a more workable self of his own" [37, p. 101]. The conscious use of self, or deliberate use of one's own responses to the patient as part of the treatment process, is regarded as a legitimate tool of O.T., and is embraced, in some form, by all O.T. frames of reference [80]. Your interpersonal effectiveness, then, becomes the critical foundation for effective treatment. Your treatment plan might be exquisite, but it will be ineffective if you lack the interpersonal therapeutic skills to implement it. Beginning communication skills were discussed in Chap. 1; however, because they are so important to treatment implementation, they are discussed here in further detail.

Noting that recent outcome studies showed no difference between types of therapy, Wills proposes that, regardless of theoretic orientation and training, therapists must be doing and accomplishing essentially similar things when they interact with patients. He suggests that there are several commonalities, or nonspecific factors, that transcend theoretic biases to account for the similar success rates among therapists [115]. Although occupational therapists do not do psychotherapy, understanding and using these commonalities may add to our ability to create the effective therapeutic relationships that are so essential to our work. Several of these factors and their influence in the therapeutic relationship follow.

Enhancement of Self-Esteem

Many people seeking help experience threats to their self-esteem; thus an important part of your relationship with the patient is to help him restore his perception of himself as a worthwhile person. The enhancement of self-esteem supplies a powerful incentive to continue therapy and helps to build commitment to the course of treatment. The value of enhanced self-esteem should not be underestimated. It has been shown to be the most prominent feature of therapy; both in effectiveness of outcome and in importance to the patient [104]. Self-esteem can be enhanced in two ways: through the therapeutic relationship, and, as O.Ts. suggest, through success at task performance.

THROUGH THE RELATIONSHIP
Effectiveness at enhancing self-esteem through the therapeutic relationship depends largely on the therapist's attitude. Liking the patient forms the foundation of

helping him feel better about himself. As mentioned previously, a number of studies suggest that the therapist's positive feelings for the patient influence the therapist's decisions about the patient's suitability for treatment and the predicted success of treatment [31]. Patients who perceive that they are not liked, respected, or treated seriously by their therapists drop out of therapy or have higher rates of unsuccessful therapy outcomes [115]. Even so, simply liking the patient is ineffective unless he knows how you feel. Your liking and respect for him can be communicated through a nonjudgmental, nonevaluative, accepting attitude [95]. This can be difficult at times, especially when the patient's behavior becomes annoying and exasperating. Patients with physical disabilities can become annoying and exasperating at times, as well, yet we often can cope with them better than a manic patient's incessant talking or a depressed patient's ceaseless complaining. Allen's exploration of the O.T. management of various psychiatric disorders provides a thought-provoking and compassionate way of understanding a whole spectrum of patient behaviors [3].

THROUGH THE TASK

Enhancing self-esteem through successful completion of a task has already been discussed in the section on "Methods" (p. 128). Although the way in which this phenomenon occurs is viewed differently by various frames of reference (either by presenting a challenge slightly above the patient's current abilities, or by reducing the novelty of the task), enhancing self-esteem through activities is seen as a major tenet of O.T. Even so, simply finding the perfect activity and giving it to your patient to complete is rarely effective. Using a task to enhance self-esteem takes several steps. First, the patient must engage in the task. You may need to encourage, facilitate, push, demonstrate, joke, praise, and so forth to get the patient started. Different patients respond to different approaches; learning which approach to use with whom comes with experience. Bing refers to this as the transference of the will from the therapist to the patient [10]. Helping the patient become involved in a task can be difficult. In most instances, your patient has the right to refuse your treatment: abide by this decision. On the other hand, one of the major symptoms of many psychiatric disorders is lack of motivation, energy, and interests [42]. Patients may refuse a task because they feel incapable of doing it, feel confused about your expectations, think the task is inappropriate or unappealing, or lack the energy to do anything. Getting your patient involved thus requires balancing these two opposing factors so that you encourage and facilitate task performance without resorting to coercion or creating resistance. At times it may feel as if you must do, as one therapist put it, "the dance of the seven veils" to get patients to participate. We know from clinical experience, however, that once patients begin to feel successful, they tend to continue in therapy. Sensitivity on your part to your approach will help keep you on the side of persuasion and motivation rather than coercion.

The second step in increasing self-esteem through task performance is to ensure successful performance. Knowing when to intervene to help the task turn out successfully will come with practical experience. For instance, if you constantly intervene to prevent errors, the patient can easily become frustrated, and you will have unwittingly reinforced his feelings of incompetence. (Perhaps the task was not structured appropriately in the first place.) On the other hand, never correcting mistakes results in a poorly executed task, which may also reinforce the patient's feelings of incompetence. There may be times when your standards of workmanship differ from those of your patient, and his proud display of a poorly done task will embarrass you. Understanding each patient's limits and abilities, the disease process, and the O.T. frames of reference provides the basis for making these challenging day-to-day decisions.

The final step is to provide positive reinforcement for task performance. Praise and encouragement must be given carefully. Enthusiastically praising a performance the patient considers unexceptional or less than his normal level can be unintentionally insulting. For example, if someone enthusiastically praised you for getting dressed, you would probably be offended. Of course you can dress yourself, you have done it since you were a child! On the other hand, lack of adequate positive encouragement can create a waning investment in the treatment process. (Why continue something for which you get no credit?) As you can see, building esteem through successful task performance is inextricably linked with your interpersonal effectiveness in the therapeutic relationship.

Modeling

Modeling has been called "the silent influence" (115, p. 386]. In a review of the literature, Wills found that a major component of therapy is the patient's perception of the therapist as a mature, competent, and admirable person whom they would like to resemble. Other studies indicate that patients tend to adopt the attitudes and values of their therapists over the course of treatment. Taken together, these studies suggest that patients in helping relationships tend to model themselves after the therapist [115]. By watching the therapist respond to life in a mature and reasonable manner, the patient may learn more constructive ways of dealing with his problematic situations. Modeling occurs whenever you are with your patient—not just when you are consciously attempting to model an alternative approach. Monitor yourself to make sure the approach you are modeling is the one you really want to encourage your patient to adopt! Not all patients seem to benefit from modeling alone [110]; however, adding demonstration, role-playing, problem solving, or projects and field trips to modeling increases its effectiveness for many patients.

Positive Expectation

"Persons who believe—for whatever reason—that they will improve or be cured tend to do just that, irrespective of whatever else is done to them" [115, p. 388]. Whether or not positive expectations affect the actual course of the disorder is not clear, but they can prevent and counteract the demoralization syndrome that frequently accompanies repeated episodes of a psychiatric disorder [97]. Patients suffering from demoralization feel hopeless, helpless, depressed (a symptom, not the DSM III Axis I diagnosis), and believe that things are not going to get better. Wills suggests that conveying a sense of hopefulness and the expectation of improvement early in therapy helps to counter demoralization [115]. Positive expectation must also be tempered with realism. Although no one knows enough yet to promise the patient that he will be cured, for many disorders (especially in the acute phase) one can realistically express confidence in the expectation of improvement in his condition. Ultimately, increasing the patient's positive expectation of improvement in a realistic manner helps sustain his strength and fights the tendency to give up. For many years, supportive treatment was considered a valuable O.T. service. Its primary objective was to help sustain the patient's strength and self-esteem during the course of the disorder and treatment through the use of activities. Supportive treatment objectives fell out of favor for many years; however, Allen proposes that we re-examine supportive treatment objectives as a viable O.T. service that we can provide to patients with acute psychiatric disorders [3].

Self-Attribution of Change

Several recent studies indicate that, because people often need to see themselves as freely determining their own behavior, changes the patient makes as a result of therapy can be more potent if the patient attributes them primarily to his own efforts rather than to those of the therapist [16,66]. Some of the recent successes of cognitive therapy techniques with depressed patients suggest that self-attribution, along with positive expectation of change, are effective weapons in fighting the patient's demoralization. Although they may not significantly alter the course of the psychiatric disorder, these weapons do seem to influence the potency of the symptoms [97]. Self-attribution of change requires increasing the patient's choices and perception of control in the therapy situation. Unless your patient believes he has some very real choices and some degree of control, he may feel coerced, resist your treatment efforts, and accomplish very little [25,98]. Both choices and opportunities for exercising control therefore must be offered to foster the patient's commitment and self-attribution of change [64].

The patient's perception of control can be increased in several ways. First, he must be given adequate information about how to exercise control in the situation, and the responsibility for doing so must not be too great. For example, asking for your patient's input in identifying goals in a specific manner (e.g., by identifying his own goals or negotiating those you selected increases his control without overwhelming him with total responsibility for the process. Unless you identify your expectations of his participation in a way he feels able to handle, it will overwhelm him, and the entire process will be counterproductive and harmful. Failure to tailor the degree of control and responsibility your patient has in the treatment situation can result in a painful, demoralizing reminder of his limitations.

Second, the patient's perception of himself as a capable person must be increased as the opportunities for control are presented. Lack of self-efficacy prevents the patient from exerting control when the opportunities arise; thus both enhancing the patient's self-esteem and increasing his opportunities and perception of control must occur together.

Finally, you need to choose the opportunities for your patient to exercise control wisely. "Increasing feelings of control when the situation is actually not controllable may have detrimental effects in the long run. . . . In such a situation, the person may make futile attempts to exert control, leading eventually to learned helplessness with its accompanying negative behavioral, cognitive, motivational, and physiological reactions" [98, p. 180]. Not only will your patient become demoralized, but your relationship will also be seriously damaged. For instance, do not suggest that the goal-setting process is mutual unless you really intend to use what your patient contributes. Solicitation of patient input without actually using what he says will quickly destroy your trustworthiness and credibility.

Development of a World View

Several studies reviewed by Beutler suggest that, over time, patients learn and develop a particular view of their own problems and of themselves as persons [9]. These views can be divided into four basic categories, or models of helping, with various degrees of implied patient responsibility for both the cause of the problem and the solution to the problem [50]. Whichever is selected affects the therapist's basic philosophy and biases the therapist toward certain frames of reference (see Table 3-1).

The moral model attributes high responsibility for both the cause of the problem and the solution to the patient, whereas the medical model attributes low responsibility for both the cause of the problem and the solution to the patient. The compensatory and enlightenment models are combinations of the moral and medical models. Lemkau, Bryant, and Brickman suggest that most clinicians and patients implicitly hold to one of these models [36]. It also appears that successful outcome of psychotherapy is related to the congruence between the viewpoints of the patient and therapist [25,36,115]. Because no conclusive evidence currently exists to indi-

*Table 3-1. The basic
models of helping, of how
a therapist views the
patient's responsibility*

Responsibility for cause of the problem	Responsibility for solution to the problem	
	High	Low
High	Moral	Enlightenment
Low	Compensatory	Medical

cate which models are most effective for various problems, one suggested approach is to determine which model the patient holds, and, at least initially, to choose the model you use accordingly [36]. On the other hand, Wills suggests that it ultimately may not matter what explanation or world view is claimed. "It may be that any coherent system that provides patients with clear rubrics for understanding their own behavior, and that of other persons, will introduce into their lives a greater degree of predictability and stability, with a consequent increase in their sense of well-being" [115, p. 396]. Whichever tack is taken, it appears that congruence between the patient's and the therapist's world views significantly relates to successful outcomes of psychotherapy [114]. We have yet to study this factor to determine how it applies to O.T. Yet, it is safe to assume that differences between the patient's and the therapist's world view can, at the minimum, create hurdles to be overcome in establishing rapport.

These "generic" factors play an important role in the development of an effective therapeutic relationship. Additionally, your personal style helps or hinders the development of a therapeutic relationship. Although there is no one right way to be, you need to be able to use your own personal qualities in an effective manner for each patient with whom you work. Ultimately, you may discover that you like working with one group of patients more than another, and that is important to know when you look for a job. For now, you need to be able to work effectively with a variety of people of different cultural, ethnic, and economic backgrounds and with a variety of problems. What a challenge!

Vary Your Approach

Every patient is different, and you need to change your approach to fit each person's needs and style. Beginning therapists frequently err on the side of being too cheerful and bubbly. A depressed patient who thinks and moves very slowly will be overwhelmed by the cheerleader approach. This is not to imply that you should be serious and glum, but rather that you should match your approach to each patient. You do not have to change your personality to be an effective therapist. There are as many effective approaches as there are therapists. Even though a slow-paced, encouraging, supportive approach may be appropriate for a depressed patient, the way you execute that approach reflects your personality and style. You can develop a repertoire of approaches that matches your personality and that works for you by observing other people, evaluating their styles, picking what seems to fit you the best, trying it out, and evaluating the results. Use the opportunities provided during your fieldwork to experiment with varying your approach to match each patient.

Self-Evaluate

After an evaluation or treatment session, take 5 minutes to sit quietly and reflect on what happened. If you can talk this over with another therapist who was present, great. In any event, you should get in the habit of reviewing each session, even if you worked alone. Use the questions listed in Fig. 3-3 to stimulate your thinking.

In retrospect, you inevitably wish you had done some things differently. (Monday-morning quarterbacks never lose the game.) On the other hand, you risk repeating errors unless you critically evaluate how you are doing. Self-evaluation not only entails pointing out your mistakes to yourself; it is also a chance to give yourself credit

Fig. 3-3. A therapist's self-assessment checklist.

At the end of each evaluation or treatment session, ask yourself the following questions:

Were the goals of the session met?

What helped or hindered reaching the goals?

What did I do that was effective? (You want to make sure you can do it again.)

What did I do that was not effective? (You want to make sure you do not do it again.)

If I were going to do this (evaluation, treatment, group) again, would I do anything differently?

Fig. 3-3. A therapist's self-assessment checklist.

for the things you do well. Growth and expertise result from learning from both your mistakes and your successes. "Expert clinicians are those who are competent in action and, simultaneously, reflect on this action to learn from it" [96, p. 616].

In summary, interpersonal effectiveness does not make up for a lack of knowledge and technical skill. The former without the latter is all show with no action. Nevertheless, you cannot be an effective therapist unless you can establish and maintain therapeutic relationships with your patients. Interpersonal effectiveness is critically important to implementing your treatment plan effectively.

Your Turn

In addition to the factors stated above, can you think of any other factor that might affect your clinical effectiveness? (Review Chap. 1 if you have trouble thinking of any.)

Evaluate Outcome

Occupational therapy is not unique in its relative lack of attention to the last critical step of the treatment process: evaluating outcome. The recent upheaval in the health care industry, however, demands accountability from the referral source for using our services and from us for showing that we were both needed and effective. Needless to say, this is a difficult task.

Careful examination of O.T.'s effectiveness in psychiatric treatment is just beginning. Linn et al. indicated that day-treatment centers offering O.T. and sustained nonthreatening environments were effective in delaying relapse and reducing some symptoms of chronic schizophrenic patients [69]. Unfortunately, the types of O.T. methods, and specific problems treated were not included in the study. Other studies have failed to demonstrate effectiveness. Small-scale comparisons of O.T. groups (both verbal and activity) with control groups have failed to demonstrate a significant difference in improvement in the patients' interpersonal communication skills [23].

One method of substantiating claims that O.T. is effective is to monitor the outcome of each treatment. The most familiar measure of outcome is a reassessment of the patient's status at discharge using the same instruments as the initial assessment. Although every therapist knows that this is an important step in the treatment process, it frequently is not done. Single-case-study research provides a feasible, practical format for systematic study of individual patient outcomes [87]. From a practical standpoint, third-party payers want to know if O.T. was needed, and if what you did benefited the patient. Systematic study of patient outcomes will satisfy this request plus add to the knowledge base about psychiatric O.T. With enough published, systematically studied outcomes, trends will appear, and hypotheses and predictions about O.T. services will become possible. Oscar Wilde reportedly said that experience is the name people give to their mistakes. It is beyond the scope of this book to teach single-case-study research methods; additional study of this area is highly recommended. Nevertheless, general principles of evaluating outcome are discussed below to help get you started.

Define Success Carefully

What would constitute a successful outcome for your patient? Outcome studies of psychotherapy are frequently categorized by a dichotomy of points of change: global or specific target symptoms [63]. In other words, success of treatment can be measured either by determining whether the specific target problem or goal was reached (e.g., increased assertiveness in making friends) or by a global measure of overall change in the person (e.g., decreased depression, increased self-esteem), or both. Other outcome studies involve measuring affective, cognitive, and behavioral changes. That is, did the patient's feelings, thoughts, or behavior change as a result of the therapy? Whichever scheme is adopted, using more than one measure of success reduces the possibility of drawing misleading conclusions because of lack of information [6, 63].

Use More Than One Measure of Outcome

Because change is multidimensional, using more than one measure of outcome reduces the chances of erroneous conclusions [6,12,63]. "It has proved far too simplistic to expect patients to show consistent and integrated improvement as a result of therapy" [63, p. 19]. For example, patients may show a marked change in the number of assertive contacts made, but report no increased comfort in these interactions. Because change occurs in different ways for each patient, multiple methods of assessing outcome provide the most reliable data [6,12,63]. Since there is no single measure of the patient's problem, different types of instruments using different sources of information yield more comprehensive data [6]. The most commonly used sources are the patient, the therapist, and instrumentation. Occasionally a trained observer or family member is also used [63]. Even though everyone focuses on the same target—the patient—data from these sources have been shown to correlate only minimally with each other. It appears that each of these sources provides different, yet valuable, pieces of information about outcome [12,63]. Your accuracy is thus increased if you tap more than one source.

Select Good Measures

What do you use to measure outcome? Should you repeat the evaluations used to assess the problem? Measures of outcome should be meaningful, sensitive, and accurate [6]. We can gain guidance for our selection from studies of psychotherapy, but, to date, no one has applied these principles to psychiatric O.T. One criterion for determining meaningfulness of the measure is the extent to which it provides information useful to the therapist. Use of the measure should provide better feedback to the therapist about the patient's progress or lack of progress than not using the measure [6,87]. Sensitivity refers to the degree to which the measure identifies minor changes in the patient. Some measures may be sensitive to weekly changes, and others may reflect global changes and be insensitive to small changes. Ideally, you would use both [6].

Accuracy refers to the measure's psychometric properties. In general, established psychometric properties enhance the measure's accuracy. Test-retest reliability and construct validity are particularly important. Unless the measure has been shown to be stable over time, any change noted can be due to the instrument and not the patient's actual change. Construct validity, or the ability of the measure to identify the presence of defined construct(s), enhances the possibility that you are measuring what you think you are measuring. Any kind of measure can be used for outcome studies. (Review the categories of instruments in Chap. 2 for ideas.) Using at least two types of instruments and at least two sources of information is suggested to minimize your chances of drawing erroneous conclusions from limited data [6].

Collect Data Before, During, and After Treatment
Certainly a measurement after treatment to compare with your assessment data is the minimal requirement. Even so, measuring outcome along the way has two major benefits. First, it gives you feedback about the effectiveness of your treatment. If it is working, you can continue, but, if it is not working, you can change gears without waiting until the end of treatment to discover that what you were doing was ineffective. Second, you have more information with which to identify the variables that affect the outcome, thus ultimately stimulating better ideas for more effective treatment [6,12].

Monitoring the effectiveness of your treatment and measuring outcome not only give you feedback so you can change your treatment accordingly, but also contribute to the knowledge base about psychiatric O.T. Single-case-study research seems a realistic way to incorporate evaluations of outcome into our daily treatment routine. Specific application of these principles to psychiatric O.T. practice is eagerly awaited.

Your Turn
Review the case example at the end of Chap. 2 and describe a plan of how you would anticipate measuring the outcome of your treatment for that patient.

Plan for Measuring Outcome
Based on your goals, define successful outcomes of treatment:

Describe outcome measures you will use (specify number, type, and names of the measures):

When will the data be collected (before, during, after therapy is completed)?

Trying It Out

The end of all thought must be action.
Aldous Huxley

This chapter has introduced you to both the planning and implementation steps of the treatment process. You learned how to write two types of goals and objectives: outcome and service. You learned how to select methods, implement treatment, and evaluate your outcomes. All that remains is to do it!

In Chap. 2, you went through the assessment process and should have ended up with a list of your patient's problems, indicators, and strengths. Starting with writing goals, continue with treatment planning. The forms you need are reprinted below for your convenience. Pay particular attention to any question or difficulty you have along the way, and note it in the space provided. These notes will identify areas that require more work.

Writing Goals and Objectives

So far, you have used a frame of reference to guide your assessment process. Using that frame of reference, which type of goals will you write: outcome or service?

At the end of Chap. 2, you prioritized the list of your patient's problems. Write a goal for each of the top two problems.

Problem   *Goal*

If You Are Writing Outcome Goals

Yes   *No*   Check your goals against the following standards:

_____ _____   Are they written as a patient performance?
_____ _____   Are they written in positive terms (something to do versus something not to do)?
_____ _____   Do they capitalize on the patient's strengths?
_____ _____   Do they have a performance, criterion, condition?
_____ _____   Do they pass the "Hey, Dad" test?
_____ _____   Are they realistic considering the time you have to work with your patient?

If You Are Writing Service Goals

Yes   *No*   Check your goals against the following standards:

_____ _____   Are they written as a therapist task?
_____ _____   Are there any hidden or implied patient performances?
_____ _____   Do the goals match your patient's cognitive level?
_____ _____   Do the goals match your patient's diagnosis?

When you are satisfied with your goals, determine whether you need objectives. If so, write them here:

Goal   *Objectives*

Yes   *No*   Check your objectives against the following standards:

——   ——   Are they measurable?
——   ——   Can they be accomplished in the time you have to work with your pa-
                   tient?
——   ——   Are they broken into steps that are realistic for your patient?

Describe your patient's involvement in goal setting:

Notes to myself:

Select Methods
Select at least three activities for each goal.

Goal:

   Activity:

   Activity:

   Activity:

Goal:

   Activity:

   Activity:

   Activity:

Yes *No* Check your activities against the following standards:

____ ____ Is the activity appropriately used with the frame of reference employed so far in the assessment and treatment-planning process? Rationale:

____ ____ Does the treatment facility have the resources for this activity? Rationale:

____ ____ If not, can the resources be found elsewhere to enable use of the activity with this patient? Rationale:

____ ____ Is the activity meaningful to the patient? Rationale:

____ ____ Is the activity appropriate for the patient's age and gender? Rationale:

____ ____ Does the activity match the problem and the goal? Rationale:

____ ____ Does the activity capitalize on the patient's strengths? Rationale:

When you are satisfied with your selection of activities, choose the structure, teaching method(s), and format.

Activity:

Structure:

Teaching Method(s):

Format:

  If group, choose the following:
    Content:

    Structure:

Activity:

Structure:

Teaching Method(s):

Format:

If group, choose the following:
  Content:

  Structure:

Rationale for selections:

Describe your patient's involvement in selecting activities:

Notes to myself:

Implementing Treatment

You are ready to go! You have planned your course of action, and now you are ready to implement it. As you have read throughout this book, self-evaluation is the key to continued professional growth. After each interaction with your patient, take a few minutes to reflect on the session and answer the following questions:

Were the goals of the session met?

What helped or hindered reaching the goals?

What did I do that was effective? (You want to make sure you can do it again.)

What did I do that was not effective? (You want to make sure you do not do it again.)

If I were going to do this (evaluation, treatment, group) again, would I do anything differently?

Notes to myself:

Evaluating Outcome

Before you get too far in your treatment, make a plan to evaluate the outcome.

Based on your goals, define successful outcomes of treatment:

Describe the outcome measures you will use (specify number, type, and names of the measures):

When will the data be collected (before, during, after therapy is completed)?

Notes to myself:

Congratulations! You have done it! You have successfully completed the entire treatment process from referral to measuring outcome—except for one very important step: documenting what you did. Few persons will know what you accomplished unless you write it down; thus, documentation is addressed in the fourth and final chapter.

1. Allen, C. K. Independence through activity: The practice of occupational therapy (psychiatry). *Am. J. Occup. Ther.* 36:731, 1982.
2. Allen, C. K. Book review: Design of rehabilitation services in psychiatric hospital settings. *Am. J. Occup. Ther.* 39:209, 1985.
3. Allen, C. K. *Occupational Therapy for Psychiatric Diseases: Measurement and Management of Cognitive Disabilities.* Boston: Little, Brown, 1985.
4. American Occupational Therapy Association. The philosophical base of occupational therapy. *Representative Assembly Resolution #531.* Rockville, MD: American Occupational Therapy Association, 1979.
5. Angel, S. L. The emotion identification group. *Am. J. Occup. Ther.* 35:256, 1981.
6. Barlow, D. H., Hayes, S. C., and Nelson, R. O. *The Scientist Practioner: Research and Accountability in Clinical and Educational Settings.* New York: Pergamon, 1984.
7. Barris, R. Environmental interactions: An extension of the model of occupation. *Am. J. Occup. Ther.* 36:637, 1982.
8. Barris, R., Kielhofner, G., and Watts, J. H. *Psychosocial Occupational Therapy: Practice in a Pluralistic Arena.* Laurel, MD: Ramsco, 1983.
9. Beutler, L. E. Convergence in counseling and psychotherapy: A current look. *Clin. Psych. Rev.* 1:79, 1981.
10. Bing, R. K. Nationally speaking: Professional nationalism *Am. J. Occup. Ther.* 37:301, 1983.
11. Blakeney, A. B, Strickland, L. R., and Wilkinson, J. H. Exploring sensory integrative dysfunction in process schizophrenia. *Am. J. Occup. Ther.* 36:399, 1983.
12. Bloom, M., and Fischer, J. *Evaluating Practice: Guidelines for the Accountable Professional.* Englewood Cliffs, NJ: Prentice-Hall, 1982.
13. Bloomer, J. S. The consumer of therapy in mental health. *Am. J. Occup. Ther.* 32:621, 1978.
14. Brady, J. P. Social skills training for psychiatric patients, I: Concepts, methods, and clinical results. *Occup. Ther. Ment. Health* 4:51, 1984.
15. Brady, J. P. Social skills training for psychiatric patients, II: Clinical outcome studies. *Occup. Ther. Ment. Health* 5:59, 1985.
16. Brehm, S. S., and Brehm, J. W. *Psychological Reactance: A Theory of Freedom and Control.* New York: Academic, 1981.
17. Charrier, G. O. Cog's Ladder: A Model of Group Development. In J. W. Pfeiffer and J. E. Jones (eds.), *Annual Handbook for Group Facilitators.* La Jolla, CA: University Associates, 1974.
18. Clark, P. N. Human development through occupation: Theoretical frameworks in contemporary occupational therapy practice, Part 1. *Am. J. Occup. Ther.* 33:505, 1979.
19. Clark, P. N. Human development through occupation: A philosophy and conceptual model for practice, Part 2. *Am. J. Occup. Ther.* 33:577, 1979.
20. Crist, P. A., Thomas, P. P., and Stone, B. L. Pre-vocational and sensorimotor training in chronic schizophrenia. *Occup. Ther. Ment. Health* 4:23, 1984.
21. Cubie, S. H., and Kaplan, K. A case analysis method for the model of human occupation. *Am. J. Occup. Ther.* 36:645, 1982.
22. Cynkin, S. *Occupational Therapy: Toward Health Through Activities.* Boston: Little, Brown, 1979.
23. DeCarlo, J. J., and Mann, W. C. The effectiveness of verbal versus activity groups in improving self-perceptions of interpersonal communication skills. *Am. J. Occup. Ther.* 39:20, 1985.
24. Denton, P. L. Teaching interpersonal skills with videotape. *Occup. Ther. Ment. Health* 2:17, 1982.
25. DiNicola, D. D., and DiMatteo, M. R. Communication, Interpersonal Influence, and Resistance to Medical Treatment. In T. A. Wills (ed.), *Basic Processes in Helping Relationships.* New York: Academic, 1982.
26. Donohue, M. V. Designing activities to develop a women's identification group. *Occup. Ther. Ment. Health* 2:1, 1982.
27. Dulay, J. L., and Steichen, M. Transitional employment for the chronically mentally ill. *Occup. Ther. Ment. Health* 2:65, 1982.
28. Duncombe, L. W., and Howe, M. C. Group work in occupational therapy: A survey of practice. *Am. J. Occup. Ther.* 39:163, 1985.
29. Falk-Kessler, J., and Froschauer, K. H. The soap opera: A dynamic group approach for psychiatric patients. *Am. J. Occup. Ther.* 32:305, 1978.

30. Falloon, I. R., and Talbot, R. E. Achieving the goals of day treatment. *J. Nerv. Ment. Dis.* 170:279, 1982.

31. Fehrenback, P. A., and O'Leary, M. R. Interpersonal Attraction and Treatment Decisions in Inpatient and Outpatient Settings. In T. A. Wills (ed.), *Basic Processes in Helping Relationships.* New York: Academic, 1982.

32. Fidler, G. S. The task-oriented group as a context for treatment. *Am. J. Occup. Ther.* 23:43, 1969.

33. Fidler, G. S. The Lifestyle Performance Profile: An Organizing Frame. In B. J. Hemphill (ed.), *The Evaluative Process in Psychiatric Occupational Therapy.* Thorofare, NJ: Slack, 1982.

34. Fidler, G. S. *Design of Rehabilitation Services in Psychiatric Hospital Settings.* Laurel, MD: Ramsco, 1984.

35. Fidler, G. S., and Fidler, J. W. Doing and becoming: Purposeful action and self actualization. *Am. J. Occup. Ther.* 32:305, 1978.

36. Fine, S. *Occupational Therapy: The Role of Rehabilitation and Purposeful Activity in Mental Health.* Rockville, MD: American Occupational Therapy Association, 1983.

37. Frank, J. D. The therapeutic use of self. *Am. J. Occup. Ther.* 12:92, 1958.

38. Frank, J. D. *Persuasion and Healing.* Baltimore: Johns Hopkins Press, 1961.

39. Gaw, B. A. Processing Questions: An Aid to Completing the Learning Cycle. In J. W. Pfeiffer and J. E. Jones (eds.), *Annual Handbook for Group Facilitators.* La Jolla, CA: University Associates, 1979.

40. Gilfoyle, E. M. Eleanor Clarke Slagle Lectureship, 1984: Transformation of a profession. *Am. J. Occup. Ther.* 38:575, 1984.

41. Goldstein, N., and Collins, T. Making videotapes: An activity for hospitalized adolescents. *Am. J. Occup. Ther.* 36:530, 1982.

42. Goodwin, D. W., and Guze, S. B. *Psychiatric Diagnosis* (3rd ed.). New York: Oxford University Press, 1984.

43. Hinojosa, J., et al. Roles and functions of the occupational therapist in the treatment of sensory integrative dysfunction. *Am. J. Occup. Ther.* 36:833, 1982.

44. Hinojosa, J., et al. Position paper: Purposeful activities. *Occupational Therapy Newspaper* February 1983, p. 5.

45. Holm, M. B. Video as a medium in occupational therapy. *Am. J. Occup. Ther.* 37:531, 1983.

46. Holmes, D. The role of the occupational therapist–work evaluator. *Am. J. Occup. Ther.* 39:308, 1985.

47. Hopkins, H. L. An Historical Perspective on Occupational Therapy. In H. L. Hopkins and H. D. Smith (eds.), *Willard and Spackman's Occupational Therapy* (5th ed.). Philadelphia: Lippincott, 1978.

48. Hurff, J. M., et al. A library skills program serving adults with mental retardation: An interdisciplinary approach. *Am. J. Occup. Ther.* 39:233, 1985.

49. Huss, A. J. From kinesiology to adaptation. *Am. J. Occup. Ther.* 35:574, 1981.

50. Karuza, J., et al. Attribution of Responsibility by Helpers and Recipients. In T. A. Wills (ed.), *Basic Processes in Helping Relationships.* New York: Academic, 1982.

51. Kaseman, B. M. Teaching money management skills to psychiatric outpatients. *Occup. Ther. Ment. Health* 1:59, 1980.

52. Kielhofner, G. (ed.) *A Model of Human Occupation: Theory and Application.* Baltimore: Williams & Wilkins, 1985.

53. Kielhofner, G., and Barris, R. Mental health occupational therapy: Trends in literature and practice. *Occup. Ther. Ment. Health.* 4:35, 1984.

54. Kielhofner, G., Burke, J. P., and Igi, C. H. A model of human occupation, Part 4: Assessment and intervention. *Am. J. Occup. Ther.* 34:777, 1980.

55. King, L. J. A sensory integrative approach to schizophrenia. *Am. J. Occup. Ther.* 28:529, 1974.

56. King, L. J. Eleanor Clarke Slagle Lectureship, 1978: Towards a science of adaptive responses. *Am. J. Occup. Ther.* 32:429, 1978.

57. King, L. J. Occupational therapy research in psychiatry: A perspective. *Am. J. Occup. Ther.* 32:15, 1978.

58. King, L. J. Occupational therapy and neuropsychiatry. *Occup. Ther. Ment. Health* 3:1, 1983.

59. Kleinman, B. L., and Bulkley, B. L. Some implications of a science of adaptive responses. *Am. J. Occup. Ther.* 36:15, 1982.

60. Kramer, L. W. SCORE: Solving community obstacles and restoring employment. *Occup. Ther. Ment. Health* 4:1, 1984.

61. Kramer, L. W., and Beidel, D. C. Job seeking skill groups: A review and application to a chronic psychiatric population. *Occup. Ther. Ment. Health* 2:37, 1982.

62. Kwako, R. Relaxation as therapy for hyperactive children. *Occup. Ther. Ment. Health* 1:29, 1980.

63. Lambert, M. J. Introduction to Assessment of Psychotherapy Outcome: Historical Perspective and Current Issues. In M. J. Lambert, E. R. Christensen, and S. S. DeJulio (eds.), *The Assessment of Psychotherapy Outcome.* New York: Wiley, 1983.

64. Lemkau, J. P., Bryant, F. B., and Brickman, P. Client Commitment to the Helping Relationship. In T. A. Wills (ed.), *Basic Processes in Helping Relationships.* New York: Academic, 1982.

65. Levy, L. L. Movement therapy for psychiatric patients. *Am. J. Occup. Ther.* 28:354, 1974.

66. Liberman, B. L. The Role of Mastery in Psychotherapy: Maintenance of Improvement and Prescriptive Change. In J. D. Frank, et al. (eds.), *Effective Ingredients of Successful Psychotherapy.* New York: Brunner/Mazil, 1978.

67. Lillie, M. D., and Armstrong, H. E. Contributions to the development of psychoeducational approaches to mental health service. *Am. J. Occup. Ther.* 36:438, 1982.

68. Lindsley, O. R. Training Parents and Teachers to Precisely Manage Children's Behavior. In M. Bloom and J. Fischer, *Evaluating Practice: Guidelines for the Accountable Professional.* Englewood Cliffs, NJ: Prentice-Hall, 1982.

69. Linn, M. W., et al. Day treatment and psychotropic drugs in the aftercare of schizophrenic patients. *Arch. Gen. Psychiatry* 36:1055, 1979.

70. Llorens, L. L. Changing balance: Environment and individual. *Am. J. Occup. Ther.* 38:29, 1984.

71. Lyons, B. G. The issue is: Purposeful versus human activity. *Am. J. Occup. Ther.* 37:493, 1983.

72. Mack, W., Lindquist, J. E., and Parham, L. D. A synthesis of occupational behavior and sensory integration concepts in theory and practice, Part 1: Theoretical foundations. *Am. J. Occup. Ther.* 36:365, 1982.

73. Mack, W., Lindquist, J. E., and Parham, L. D. A synthesis of occupational behavior and sensory integration concepts in theory and practice, Part 2: Clinical applications. *Am. J. Occup. Ther.* 36:433, 1982.

74. Mager, R. F. *Preparing Instructional Objectives* (2nd ed.). Belmont, CA: Fearon, 1962.

75. Mager, R. F. *Goal Analysis.* Belmont, CA: Fearon, 1972.

76. Miller, K. J. Music for movement. *Mental Health Special Interest Section Newsletter.* 6:1, 1983.

77. Moriarity, B. E. Successful goal planning with the mentally disabled. *Soc. Rehabil. Record* 1:3, 1974.

78. Mosey, A. C. The concept and use of developmental groups. *Am. J. Occup. Ther.* 24:272, 1970.

79. Mosey, A. C. *Three Frames of Reference for Mental Health.* Thorofare, NJ: Slack, 1970.

80. Mosey, A. C. *Occupational Therapy: Configuration of A Profession.* New York: Raven, 1981.

81. Mueller, S., and Suto, M. Starting a stress management programme. *Mental Health Special Interest Section Newsletter* 6(2):1, 1983.

82. Mumford, M. S. A comparison of verbal and activity groups. *Am. J. Occup. Ther.* 28:281, 1974.

83. Neistadt, M. E., and Marques, K. An independent living skills training program. *Am. J. Occup. Ther.* 38:671, 1984.

84. Nelville, A. The model of human occupation and depression. *Mental Health Special Interest Section Newsletter* 8(1):1, 1985.

85. Oakley, F., Kielhofner, G., and Barris, R. An occupational therapy approach to assessing psychiatric patients' adaptive functioning. *Am. J. Occup. Ther.* 39:147, 1985.

86. Orgren, K. A living skills program in an acute psychiatric setting. *Mental Health Special Interest Section Newsletter* 6(4):1, 1983.

87. Ottenbacher, K., and York, J. Strategies for evaluating clinical change: Implications for practice and research. *Am. J. Occup. Ther.* 38:647, 1984.

88. Palmer, F., and Gatti, D. Transitional employment project. *Occup. Ther. Ment. Health* 2:23, 1982.

89. Palmer, F., and Gatti, D. Vocational treatment model. *Occup. Ther. Ment. Health* 5:41, 1985.

90. Posthuma, B. W. Sensory integration in mental health: Dialogue with Lorna Jean King. *Occup. Ther. Ment. Health* 3:1, 1983.

91. Rance, C., and Price, A. Poetry as a group project. *Am. J. Occup. Ther.* 27:239, 1973.

92. Reed, K. L., and Sanderson, S. R. *Concepts of Occupational Therapy* (2nd ed.). Baltimore: Williams & Wilkins, 1983.

93. Reilly, M. Eleanor Clarke Slagle Lectureship, 1962: Occupational Therapy Can Be One of the Great Ideas of 20th Century Medicine. *Am. J. Occup. Ther.* 16:1, 1962.

94. Rider, B. A. Sensorimotor treatment of chronic schizophrenics. *Am. J. Occup. Ther.* 32:451, 1978.

95. Rogers, J. C. The spirit of independence: The evolution of a philosophy. *Am. J. Occup. Ther.* 36:709, 1982.

96. Rogers, J. C. Eleanor Clarke Slagle Lectureship, 1983: Clinical reasoning: The ethics, science, and art. *Am. J. Occup. Ther.* 37:601, 1983.

97. Rotzer, F. T., Koch, H., and Pflug, B. A Cognitive–Behavioral Treatment Programme for Depressed Outpatients. In J. D. Williams (ed.), *The Psychological Treatment of Depression.* New York: Free Press, 1984.

98. Schorr, D., and Rodin, J. The Role of Perceived Control in Practitioner–Patient Relationships. In T. A. Wills (ed.), *Basic Processes in Helping Relationships.* New York: Academic, 1982.

99. Schroeder, C. V., et al. *SBC Adult Psychiatric Sensory Integration Evaluation Manual.* La Jolla, CA: SBC Research Associates, 1978.

100. Schroeder, C. V., et al. The Adult Psychiatric Sensory Integration Evaluation. In B. J. Hemphill (ed.), *The Evaluative Process in Psychiatric Occupational Therapy.* Thorofare, NJ: Slack, 1982.

101. Schwartzberg, S. L., Howe, M. C., and McDermott, A. A comparison of three treatment group formats for facilitating social interaction. *Occup. Ther. Ment. Health* 2:1, 1982.

102. Scott, A. H., and Haggarty, E. J. Structuring goals via goal attainment scaling in occupational therapy groups in a partial hospitalization setting. *Occup. Ther. Ment. Health* 4:39, 1984.

103. Shannon, P. D., and Snortum, J. R. An activity group's role. *Am. J. Occup. Ther.* 19:334, 1965.

104. Smith, M. L., et al. *The Benefits of Psychotherapy.* Baltimore: Johns Hopkins Press, 1980.

105. Sparling, J. W., and Mitchell, M. M. Use of taxonomies to sequence clinical objectives. *Am. J. Occup. Ther.* 36:388, 1982.

106. Strupp, H. H., and Hadley, S. W. Specific vs nonspecific factors in psychotherapy: A controlled study of outcome. *Arch. Gen. Psychiatry* 36:1125, 1979.

107. Talbot, J. F. An inpatient adolescent living skills program. *Occup. Ther. Ment. Health* 3:35, 1983.

108. Thomes, L. J., and Bajema, S. L. The life skills development program: A history, overview, and update. *Occup. Ther. Ment. Health* 3:35, 1983.

109. Tiffany, E. G. Psychiatry and Mental Health. In H. L. Hopkins and H. D. Smith (eds.), *Willard and Spackman's Occupational Therapy* (5th ed.). New York: Lippincott, 1978.

110. Walter, G. A., and Marks, S. E. *Experiential Learning and Change: Theory, Design and Practice.* New York: Wiley, 1981.

111. Watson, M. R., and Thomes, L. J. Project ABLE: A model for management of stress in the army soldier. *Occup. Ther. Ment. Health* 3:55, 1983.

112. West, W. L. Historical Perspectives. In *Occupational Therapy: 2001 AD.* Rockville, MD: American Occupational Therapy Association, 1979.

113. West, W. L. A reaffirmed philosophy and practice of occupational therapy for the 1980s. *Am. J. Occup. Ther.* 38:15, 1984.

114. Wills, T. A. Directions for Research on Helping Relationships. In T. A. Wills (ed.), *Basic Processes in Helping Relationships.* New York: Academic, 1982.

115. Wills, T. A. Nonspecific Factors in Helping Relationships. In T. A. Wills (ed.), *Basic Processes in Helping Relationships.* New York: Academic, 1982.

116. Yerxa, E. The Philosophical Base of Occupational Therapy. In *Occupational Therapy: 2001 AD.* Rockville, MD: American Occupational Therapy Association, 1979.

Documentation

"When *I* use a word," Humpty Dumpty said, in rather a scornful tone, "it means just what I choose it to mean—neither more nor less."

Lewis Carroll
Through the Looking-Glass

Jo had done it! She had completed Mr. Smithson's interview, assessment, and treatment plan. She felt good about how she had done, considering that he was her first patient. Now she had to write her findings in a note. As she threw her third rewrite into the wastebasket, Jo wondered if she would ever get the note written. *What am I going to do if writing notes always takes me this long?* she thought. *I'll never get home in time for dinner!* It seemed to Jo that she had too much information, but she could not decide what to include and what to leave out. *Am I writing stuff that everybody already knows?* she wondered. *How do I organize all of this so it makes sense?*

Jo's struggle with writing notes is familiar. Documentation is not a favorite task of many clinicians. It is difficult to shift gears at the end of a busy day to write notes, yet documentation is a critical component of the job. During the course of the day, you document many types of information, such as patient attendance, supplies needed, charges and statistics, and use of your time. This chapter addresses only reports of direct patient treatment: patient notes.

Background Information

In general, notes have two major functions. First, they are a major avenue of communication between you and the other team members. Regardless of what you actually accomplished with the patient, your notes are the only evidence of what happened. You may not always have the opportunity to share your information about the patient in person. Writing a note thus increases the chances that all staff members will receive your information. This point cannot be stressed too strongly. Much of O.T.'s interdisciplinary credibility is gained through the notes therapists write. Timely, concise, and relevant notes help you gain respect from other team members (assuming the treatment you delivered was appropriate and useful). Notes also document the services you provided to the patient for regulatory and payment purposes. Notes are reviewed for many reasons, usually after the patient has been discontinued from O.T. Notes are reviewed for quality-assurance studies, such as determining the length of time between referral and treatment, the adequacy of the assesment and treatment delivered to a particular patient, and the timeliness and quality of notes. Notes are reviewed by reimbursement sources to determine if O.T. was needed, what services were provided and why, and the patient's response to the treatment. Your degree of compliance with the institution's note-writing policy for both regulatory and legal purposes is derived from your notes. Rarely will you be given the opportunity to elaborate on any of these issues in person; thus, failure to document in a comprehensive and timely manner can carry severe financial, legal, and ethical consequences. Note writing requires juggling the conciseness and timeliness needed for staff communication (long notes are generally not read) with the comprehensiveness needed to document adequately and the limited time you have to write notes each day. This task becomes easier as you gain experience. For now, you are learning a new skill; try not to be discouraged if it takes you longer than you think it should. Your fieldwork experience will provide you with many opportunities to develop good documentation habits that will serve you well whatever your speciality area.

Hints for Better Notes

Each facility has its own protocol for writing notes, as you will learn in your fieldwork and on the job. However, there are a few basic rules that can help you sharpen your notes. The first and most important is: be concise. Long notes simply are not read, thus defeating one of the purposes of writing a note in the first place. Use good grammar and spelling. As mentioned before, much of O.T.'s interdisciplinary credibility comes from the notes therapists write. Grammar and spelling errors imply sloppiness and are both unprofessional and inexcusable. Refer to yourself as "this writer," "this student," or "this therapist." It gives a more formal, professional tone to the note. Regardless of what other staff members do, write legibly! If your handwriting cannot be deciphered, the note is useless, and you have wasted your time. Each note should be dated and signed with your full name and title: OTS or OTR. If you make a mistake while writing a note, draw a line through the word so that one can still read what it says, and write "(error)" and the corrected word immediately following. For example:

Mr. Smithson scored ~~120~~(error) 140 on the . . .

This method of correcting mistakes is a legal protection; it ensures that the notes cannot be altered after they are written. Never use white correction fluid or black out the mistaken work so completely that it cannot be read. Finally, for the same legal reasons, use a pen not a pencil to write notes. Check your notes for these points using the guide provided (Fig. 4-1).

Types of Notes

As mentioned previously, each facility has its own format and protocol for writing notes. The following information illustrates general principles that can help you get started. Basically, you will be asked to write four types of patient notes: referral, initial, progress, and discharge. The content of the notes reflects the work you have already done with the patient.

Referral Notes

As you recall from Chap. 2, referral notes are needed if there is a delay in screening (usually beyond 48 hours). Following are three examples of referral notes documenting different reasons for the delay in receiving O.T. services.

Example 1: Patient Unavailable Due to Testing

July 3, 1985. This 24-year-old female with a diagnosis of schizo-affective disorder was referred to O.T. on June 30, 1985, by Dr. Freud for evaluation and treatment of basic life skills. Patient has been scheduled for numerous diagnostic tests at times conflicting with the O.T. schedule. Initial contact with patient has been made. O.T. screening will be delayed until completion of the medical work-up on July 5, 1985. Jo Rabson, OTS, Terry Brown, OTR.

Fig. 4-1. Checklist for notewriting.

		Check each of your notes for the following format points:

Yes	No	
____	____	Are all the important data included?
____	____	Is the note as concise as I can make it?
____	____	Are the grammar and spelling accurate?
____	____	Did I refer to myself in the third person?
____	____	Is it legible?
____	____	Is it dated?
____	____	Is it signed?
____	____	Are the errors corrected accurately?

Example 2: Patient Refuses to Attend

July 3, 1985. This 45-year-old male with diagnosis of major depressive episode was referred to O.T. on July 1, 1985, by Dr. Freud for evaluation of task performance. Patient has been contacted daily and refuses either to attend O.T. or to participate in evaluation on the unit. Physician has been notified. Case will be kept open and daily contacts made to encourage patient to participate. Jo Rabson, OTS, Terry Brown, OTR.

Example 3: Responding to Inappropriate Referral

July 3, 1985. This 85-year-old female with diagnosis of Alzheimer's disease was referred to O.T. on July 1, 1985, by Dr. Freud for self-awareness activities. Her cognitive impairment counterindicates participation in this group. Nevertheless, she could benefit from evaluation of her cognitive status for potential grave disability, and supportive routine tasks. Physician has been notified; verbal referral received to proceed with above recommendation. O.T. screening to be completed by July 5, 1985. Jo Rabson, OTS, Terry Brown, OTR.

In summary, referral notes are a brief record that the referral was received and an indication of your intention to follow through with the request made. In actual practice, these notes seem to be read most often by chart auditors, not by other team members. They occasionally need to be written, but they are not worth a lot of creative effort.

Initial Notes

Initial notes are the formal record of your assessment and treatment plan; thus almost all the information you gathered in Chaps. 2 and 3 needs to appear in this note. Obviously, you must be selective. Each facility uses its own format for writing notes. Generally, however, the information is organized into three basic categories: data, interpretation, and plan—the facts, what they mean, and what you plan to do about it. This format is used for all notes except referral notes. Initial note information is organized as follows:

Category	Information included
Data	Results of screening interview and performance assessment; observations of patient during screening or evaluation; additional evaluations used (title, numeric score [if any], what score means)
Interpretation	Problems and problem indicators; strengths
Plan	Goals; objectives; methods (activity and format)

The chart review, which you completed in Chap. 2, is not included in the initial note. That information was for your use to help determine the appropriate treatment for the patient. It would be redundant to write it again. You probably also noticed that not all of the methods are included in this note. The structure, teaching methods, and content/structure of the group are important for O.T., but usually not of interest to other professionals. Nevertheless, there are three good reasons why it is important to take the time to plan the methods as described in the last chapter. First, it will improve your treatment. Vague plans lead to vague treatment. If you are not sure exactly what you are going to do with a patient, it probably will not get done. Second, if the methods are written down in detail and kept in the O.T. department (perhaps on the back of the chart review card), it will be easier for another therapist to cover for your patient when you are not there. Finally, writing down methods in detail records what you did with a particular patient. Although you may find it hard to believe that you could forget something like that, having this information at your fingertips will facilitate your self-evaluation and clinical growth.

Basically, the initial note documents the patient's functioning in specified situations (e.g., interview, evaluation, and O.T. clinic), interprets what the information means, and specifies the plan of action. As you learned in Chaps. 2 and 3, this information all matches. The problems are prioritized, and the most important problem has a corresponding goal(s). The other problems are addressed later, and a brief statement to that effect is included in the note. If necessary, the goal is broken down into objectives, and the methods selected directly address the problem and the goal. Initial notes for the examples used in the last two chapters follow. These examples are presented only to illustrate the format for note writing and are *not* intended to guide the O.T. treatment of actual patients. As you have learned, treatment must be tailored to each patient.

Example 1: Functional Performance

Initial Note. July 30, 1984.

Data. This 14-year-old male patient with diagnosis of adolescent avoidant disorder was referred to O.T. by Dr. Freud on July 29, 1985. He was interviewed and evaluated using the Adolescent Role Survey and the Comprehensive Occupational Therapy Evaluation (COTE) on July 29. During the interview, the patient reported that "I'm not as good as the other kids" and stated that his goals for treatment were to "learn how to make friends" and to "feel better about myself." The Adolescent Role Survey indicated that the patient has no good friends and spends all of his leisure time alone. He reports no involvement in extracurricular activities at school. Patient has several interests that could provide contacts with peers (movies, fishing, model planes). Patient reports good relations with his family. The COTE (structured observation of group activity) indicated that patient's task skills were not problematic. Nevertheless, he did not initiate interaction with other group members and responded only when the therapist addressed him directly. He was observed to make five negative self-statements during the 1-hour group, and he was asked to self-monitor the number of negative self-statements during the following two O.T. sessions. He reported four during an individual session and six during a group session. Both reports were corroborated by this therapist.

Interpretation. Patient's problems relevant to O.T. appear to be: 1) feels inferior to peers, as indicated by lack of contact with peers over the past 6 months and high number of negative self-statements, and 2) not assertive in making friends, as indicated by his lack of initiating contact with peers. Patient's strengths include various interests that can provide contact with peers, valuing of friendships, and unimpaired task skills. Patient also continues to attend school regularly and is maintaining a B–C average.

Plan. Goal: Patient is to attend movie with peers two times in the next month.
    Objective: By August 8, patient is to make contact with two peers.
    Objective: By August 15, patient is to attend movie with peers.
    Methods: *Activity*—social skills
              Format—group

Only the first problem will be addressed at this time. Patient is to be reassessed at the end of the month. Patient is to attend O.T. three times per week (M, W, F) after school. Jo Rabson, OTS and Susan Smith, OTR.

In this example, the screening was completed right away, so the referral information was included in the initial note, and no referral note was needed.

Example 2: Sensory Integration

Initial Note. July 30, 1985.

Data. Patient was interviewed and evaluated using the Schroeder, Block, and Campbell instrument (SBC) on July 29, 1985. During the interview, patient reported being told she was "slow in developing" and that she had considerable difficulty learning to ride a bike. Family history indicates one sister with learning disorder and a maternal aunt diagnosed with schizophrenia. Patient states one major problem at this time is her lack of balance; this is most notable when she tries to enter and leave the city bus (primary mode of transportation). She reports that she has fallen several times resulting in lack of willingness to use the bus system. SBC results indicate scores of 4 (highly dysfunctional) on the Romberg and Classical Romberg subtests; protective extension was elicited in 3/4 trials indicating possible dysfunction in this area. Patient's sitting balance and overall muscle strength are not problematic.

Interpretation. Patient's primary problem relevant to O.T. appears to be impaired balance as evidenced by failure to perform Romberg in 4/4 trials or to hold the sharpened Romberg for 10 seconds. Patient's strengths include good strength, sitting balance, and desire to improve balance enough to allow her to use the bus.

Plan. Goal: Patient is to perform Romberg with no difficulty in 4/4 trials and to hold the sharpened Romberg for 30 seconds in the next 6 weeks.
　　　Methods: *Activity*—gross motor balancing activities
　　　　　　　Format—individual sessions

Patient's postural reflexes will be assessed further. Patient's functioning will be reassessed in 3 weeks to determine status. Group movement activities will be considered at that time. Patient is to attend O.T. three times per week (M, T, F) from 9:00–10:00 A.M. Jo Rabson, OTS and Susan Smith, OTR.

Because the screening was delayed with this patient, a referral note had already been written, and no referral information was needed in this note. This note also illustrates how to include your intention to assess a particular area of functioning further (postural reflexes).

Example 3: Model of Human Occupation

Initial Note: July 30, 1985

Data: This 42-year-old female with diagnosis of dysthymic disorder was referred to O.T. by Dr. Freud on July 28, 1985. She was interviewed and evaluated using the Role Checklist, Leisure Interest Checklist, and observation in individual O.T. activities on July 28 and 29, 1985. During the interview, the patient stated, "I always seem to be busy taking care of everyone else and don't do the things I want to do." Interview and Role Checklist indicated patient's primary current roles are care giver, home maintainer, volunteer, family member, religious participant, friend, and participant in organizations. She rated all of these as highly valued roles, but stated she has had difficulty "motivating myself" to participate in many of these roles in the past month. She stated that she never had difficulty "managing her time" or "feeling fulfilled" prior to this past month. In addition, she rated hobbyist/amateur as a highly valued role, but she is not currently participating in this role. The Leisure Interest Checklist indicated several occupations of interest to the patient (quilting, planting terrariums, macrame). She stated that she used to feel competent in her life, but lately she has not been satisfied with her ability to perform adequately in any of her roles. "I don't feel like I'm doing anything well." Observation of the patient in the O.T. clinic indicated no impairment in her performance skills.

Interpretation. Patient's primary problems relevant to O.T. appear to be an imbalance in her current role performance as indicated by low satisfaction with her role performance and the discrepancy between valued roles (hobbyist/amateur) and lack of current participation in that role. Her strengths include a variety of valued roles and a history of successful role performance.

Plan: Goal: Patient is to participate in two activities of valued role (hobbyist/amateur) in the next 2 weeks.
　　　Methods: *Activity*—quilting and planting terrariums
　　　　　　　Format—individual and group

Patient's role performance will be assessed. Patient is to attend O.T. daily from 10:00–11:00 A.M. for individual treatment sessions for 1 week. Patient's status will be reassessed at that time and group activities considered. Jo Rabson, OTS and Susan Smith, OTR.

This example illustrates how to use the patient's statements (subjective data) in your notes. Note that "patient states that she feels" is used rather than "patient feels." You cannot really know how she feels; you can only state what she told you about how she feels.

Example 4: Cognitive Disabilities

Initial Note. July 30, 1985

Data. This 21-year-old male with a diagnosis of schizo-affective disorder was referred to O.T. by Dr. Freud on July 30, 1985. He was interviewed and screened using the Allen Cognitive Level Test and observations of an individual activity. During the interview, patient reported that his highest level of functioning was in the spring of 1984, when he was attending college and living in a dormatory. He completed the fall semester, but started to have difficulty in the spring and dropped out of school. Patient has worked for father on the farm when not attending school, but has never worked at competitive employment. Both patient and father report that relationship is strained. This is the third hospitalization in the past 18 months, and patient has been unable to complete a semester at school successfully since 1984. Currently, patient exhibits blunted affect, irritability, and paranoid delusions (states others in the room are thinking "bad thoughts" about him). The Allen Cognitive Level Test and observations of his performance on an individual activity indicate that he is currently functioning at cognitive level 4, indicating difficulty with attention, new learning, and ability to correct errors. Patient is aware of his symptoms and will apologize for his irritable behavior, but denies limitations in performance capabilities. He states his goals are to return to school and to become an engineer.

Interpretation. Patient's primary problems relevant to O.T. are that he appears to be unable to: 1) invent new motor actions, as evidenced by his failure to correct errors when they are pointed out and he is given demonstrated solutions (state that he likes it that way) and his inability to remember two-step directions, and 2) sustain attention. His attention span is limited to the immediate, as demonstrated by his inability to sustain attention and interest in his project beyond two sessions. Patient's strengths include interest in activities, awareness of a goal, and a desire to reach it. Although patient is visibly uncomfortable in interactions with therapist, he asks for and follows directions from therapist to complete the goal.

Plan. Goals: 1) Provide short-term tasks and assist with patient problem solving to monitor functional ability and symptoms.
2) Monitor cognitive level through task performance as neuroleptic medication is titrated.
Methods: *Activity*—basic skills review group and basic crafts
Format—individual sessions and group as tolerated

Patient is to attend O.T. twice a day, at 11:00 A.M. and 2:00 P.M. Patient's status will be reviewed every 2 days. Jo Rabson, OTS and Susan Smith, OTR.

Although you generally do not rewrite information in your note that would appear elsewhere in the chart, selected examples may be included, as in the preceding note, if they are relevant to the information you are presenting.

In summary, the initial note documents your assessment, interprets what it means, and states your plan of action for treatment. You probably also noticed that each of the notes contained a schedule for O.T. treatment sessions. This schedule should appear in the initial note; it will help other team members with scheduling appointments. The frequency and length of treatment are based on clinical judgment. Until more clinical outcome studies can be performed to indicate how long treatment for specific problems should take, you will have to rely on your clinical supervisor to help you make a realistic schedule.

Your Turn

In the last two chapters, you followed four problems through the sequence of identifying problem indicators, goals, objectives, and methods. Choose one of these examples and write the information you have already gathered into an initial note. You will need to make up some information, but the primary purpose of this exercise is to help you organize the information in the right format. Accuracy of content will be considered in the notes you write at the end of the chapter. For now, consider this exercise a good review of the information you have learned. The frame of reference is already identified for each example, but you need to decide:

Type of treatment facility and expected length of treatment.
Patient's age and diagnosis.
Screening and evaluation instruments used in the assessment.
Numeric score on instrument (if any) and what it means.
Treatment schedule.

Initial Note

Date:

Data:

Interpretation:

Plan:

Signature:

When actually planning treatment for a patient, you start at the beginning and run through the entire sequence, including screening, evaluation, problem identification, goals, and methods. Although this exercise asked you to skip the first steps of the process, you can use it to determine your command of those steps. Use the checklist in Figs. 4-1 and 4-2 to review your note and share your results with a fellow student or colleague. The more feedback you receive, the more efficient and accurate your notes will become.

Fig. 4-2. *Initial note checklist.*

Check your initial note to see if you have included the following:

Yes No

_____ _____ Referral data (if no referral note was written)
_____ _____ Date and type of evaluation(s) given
_____ _____ Results of interview, evaluations
_____ _____ What these results mean
_____ _____ Observations of patient during screening and evaluation
_____ _____ Patient's problems and problem indicators
_____ _____ Patient's strengths
_____ _____ Goals and objectives
_____ _____ Methods (activities, format)
_____ _____ Additional information needed (e.g., follow-up evaluation, delay in working on some problems)
_____ _____ O.T. schedule including date of reassessment

Progress Notes

Progress notes are an ongoing record of your treatment and the patient's status. They follow the same basic organizational categories as initial notes:

Category	Information included
Data	Patient's attendance at O.T.; O.T. treatment given; reevaluation of patient's status (names of instruments used, numeric score [if any], what score means); observations of patient; relevant patient comments
Interpretation	Changes in patient status from initial evaluation to present; therapist's opinion about the meaning of data collected so far
Plan	Plan for O.T. treatment (continue previous plan, add new components, delete old components)

As with initial notes, you will have a lot of information that needs to be condensed for progress notes, and you will have to be selective about what you include.

Each facility determines the procedures specifying how often progress notes must be written. In some instances, such as when treatment is prolonged, you may write several progress notes on the same patient. Other situations will require only one note. It is your responsibility to keep track of when your notes are due and to make sure they are done on time. Note that the time frames of these progress notes follow the plan specified in the initial note. Some examples of progress notes follow:

Example 1: Functional Performance

Progress Note. August 13, 1985

Data. Patient has attended O.T. six times in the past 2 weeks and participated in a social skills group. Patient has initiated contact with other group members and reports having initiated short contacts with peers at school. He has been observed to respond to contacts from other group members and to hold 5- to 7-minute conversations without therapist present. The number of negative self-statements has decreased to average two per group. Patient has not attended movie with peers yet, stating, "I don't know how to do it."

Interpretation. Patient has made progress in both initiating contact and responding to others since initial evaluation. In addition, his negative self-statements have been reduced by about half. Continues to have difficulty taking risks with peers, particularly peers at school. It appears, however, that practicing with other group members is an effective strategy for increasing his confidence to attempt interaction with peers at schol.

Plan. Continue previous plan with additional objective and the following modification of dates for completing objectives:

> Objective: By August 20, patient is to initiate group activity of attending movie with other group members.
>
> Objective: By August 30, patient is to attend one movie with school peer(s).

Methods and O.T. schedule remain the same. Jo Rabson, OTS and Susan Smith, OTR.

Example 2: Sensory Integration

Progress Note. August 20, 1985

Data. Patient has attended O.T. nine times in the past 3 weeks and has participated in gross motor activities focused on improving balance. Patient's postural reflexes (protective extension, tonic labyrinthine, asymmetric tonic neck, and symmetric tonic neck) were evaluated on August 18, 1985; no difficulty was noted. Re-evaluation of overall functioning with the SBC indicates scores of 3 on both the Romberg and the Classical Romberg (indicating continued dysfunction). Patient states that she enjoys the activities and that she can notice an improvement. Continues to be afraid to use city bus.

Interpretation. Patient's balance shows improvement both in formal evaluation and in clinical observations. At current level, she may be able to manage the bus safely; however, her anxiety about falling limits her willingness to try this independently.

Plan.
1) Reduce individual sessions to two sessions per week (Monday, Friday).
2) Add movement group (Tuesday).
3) Assess patient's functioning on actual bus ride to determine if other factors need to be addressed.

Jo Rabson, OTS and Susan Smith, OTR.

Example 3: Model of Human Occupation

Progress Note: August 6, 1985

Data. Patient has attended O.T. five times in past week and has begun one activity and stated that "it's easier than I thought it would be." Patient has had difficulty motivating herself to attend O.T.; she initially declines, but will attend if encouraged. Once in the clinic, she becomes engaged in the activity and works for the entire 1-hour period. Observation was shared with patient, and she agreed that for the past month it has been "hard for me to get going at something." She stated that she felt much better when she was doing something, and "I just need to get a push to get started."

Interpretation. Patient is beginning to experience success at activity in valued role, but no overall change in status has been observed.

Plan. Continue with previous plan with the following additions:
1) Women's group three times a week (M, W, F) 3:00–4:00 P.M.
2) Individual activities done in basic crafts group 9:00–10:00 A.M. daily.
3) Evaluation of time management skills.

Jo Rabson, OTS and Susan Smith, OTR

Example 4: Cognitive Disabilities

Progress Note. August 1, 1985

Data. Patient has attended two Basic Skills groups and two individual sessions this week. He continues to be irritable and is easily distracted by stimulation. Patient appeared groggy this morning and was unable to stay awake during O.T. group. His gait was unsteady, and gross motor coordination was impaired. When asked how he was doing 1 hour after group, he stated, "I never got to come to O.T. this morning. I lost the whole morning."

Interpretation. No change in cognitive status noted; attention and ability to notice and correct errors remain impaired. Patient appeared to be having an undesirable reaction to his medication this morning. Physician and contact nurse were notified of this observation.

Plan. Continue previous plan. Continue to observe for changes in functioning as medication is titrated. Reassess in 2 days. Jo Rabson, OTS and Susan Smith, OTR.

In summary, progress notes record your ongoing treatment, the patient's responses and status, your opinion of what that means, and your plan of action. Strive to make them short and to the point. Frequently beginning therapists think that progress must be demonstrated because the note is called a progress note. As the preceding examples illustrate, this just is not always possible. The note needs to reflect what you really did and the patient's current status, even if no progress is demonstrated. Such circumstances behoove you to re-evaluate your program to see if you are on the right track, or if there is some other explanation for why progress has not been made. Professional conduct mandates that the content of the note be accurate and truthful, even when you are not satisfied with the results you have to report.

Your Turn

Write a progress note for the ongoing treatment of the patient you used in the last exercise. Because we have no information on the treatment of this patient, this note is based on purely hypothetic data. The purpose of this exercise is to help you learn the format for writing progress notes; accuracy of content is covered at the end of the chapter.

Progress Note

Date:

Data:

Interpretation:

Plan:

Signature:

Use the checklists in Figs. 4-1 and 4-3 to make sure that all the pertinent information is included. Your note-writing skills will improve by sharing this note with a fellow student or colleague and asking for feedback. Collaboration and constructive criticism are skills that will help you grow professionally; sharing this note is a good place to start.

Discharge Summaries

The final type of note is a discharge summary written when the patient is discontinued from O.T. treatment. This note uses the same basic format as the other two notes:

Fig. 4-3. Progress note checklist.

Check your progress notes to see if you have included the following:

Yes	No	
___	___	Patient attendance at O.T.
___	___	O.T. treatment given
___	___	Results of further evaluation or re-evaluation
___	___	Relevant observations of patient during O.T.
___	___	Changes in patient status
___	___	Your interpretation of what this information means
___	___	Plan for treatment (additions, deletions, remain the same)

Category	Information included
Data	Introductory data (date of referral to O.T., reason for referral, number of times seen in O.T.); patient's status at beginning of treatment (specific problems and problem indicators); goals of O.T. treatment; types of methods used; patient's status at discharge, including progress on specific problems noted at beginning of treatment
Interpretation	Therapist's opinion about what above data mean
Plan	Additional recommendations (e.g., home program, community contacts)

This note does not have to be a detailed description of the entire course of the patient's treatment. It should be as concise and to the point as the other notes have been. Yet discharge summaries are often the only notes that third-party payers read. Payment can be denied if the assessment, treatment plan, treatment implementation, and results are not adequately documented. Examples of discharge summaries follow:

Example 1: Functional Performance

Discharge Summary. September 13, 1985

Data. Patient was referred to O.T. on July 28, 1985, for social skills training. He was seen 15 times. At beginning of treatment, patient's problems were identified as: 1) feels inferior to peers, as indicated by lack of contact with peers over the past 6 months and high number of negative self-statements, and 2) not assertive in making friends, as indicated by his lack of initiative in contacting peers in the past month. Goals of O.T. were for patient to attend two movies with school peers during course of treatment. Methods used included social skills training, both individual and group. At discharge, patient had met the goal. He also organized a trip to the movies with the social skills group, and the number of negative self-statements decreased with only an occasional comment recorded.

Interpretation. Patient made significant improvements in social skills during the course of treatment. Although decreasing negative self-statements was not a direct treatment goal, it occurred as the patient gained more confidence in his social skills. Treatment methods that seemed the most effective were role playing and practice with social skills group before attempting interactions with school peers.

Plan. Discontinue patient from O.T. Recommend home program of periodic review of social skills information when he encounters unfamiliar situations. Recommend involvement in extracurricular group (of patient's choice) at school, which would keep him involved with peers. Jo Rabson, OTS and Susan Smith, OTR.

Example 2: Sensory Integration

Discharge Summary. September 24, 1985

Data. Patient was referred to O.T. on July 29, 1985, for assessment and treatment of sensorimotor dysfunction. She was seen by O.T. 24 times. At beginning of treatment, patient's primary problem relevant to O.T. treatment was impaired balance, as indicated by failure on Romberg and Classical Romberg tests. The O.T. goal was for patient to be able to perform both of these tests without dysfunction. Treatment methods included both individual and group gross motor activities, ranging from standing balance to maintaining balance when moving and attention was distracted. At discharge, patient had successfully completed the goal. Re-evaluation with the Romberg and Classical Romberg indicated no dysfunction. At discharge, she was functionally able to enter and exit the city bus.

Interpretation. Patient's balance improved significantly. Functionally, she gained greater independence with the ability to use the city bus without anxiety about falling.

Plan. Discontinue patient from O.T. Recommend patient join YWCA's "Exercise for Nonexercisers" group for continued gross motor activities. Jo Rabson, OTS and Susan Smith, OTR.

Example 3: Model of Human Occupation

Discharge Summary. August 13, 1985

Data. Patient was referred to O.T. on July 28, 1985, for assessment and treatment of role dysfunction. She was seen 10 times. At beginning of treatment, patient's problem relevant to O.T. was identified as an imbalance in her current role performance, as indicated by low satisfaction with her role performance and a discrepancy between a valued role (hobbyist/amateur) and lack of current participation in that role. O.T. goal was for patient to participate in two activities of this valued role in the 2-week treatment period. Treatment methods included individual activities of patient's choice in both individual and group sessions, and a women's group. At discharge, patient had completed two activities and started a third. Patient expressed satisfaction with her achievements and stated she felt "good that I did something for myself for a change." Patient's energy level and initiative to attend O.T. were observed to improve by discharge.

Interpretation. At discharge, patient was expressing more satisfaction with abilities and involvement in hobbyist role. She identified time management as an issue that needed additional work. The women's group was an effective method, and patient has made a commitment to continue with a similar group in the outpatient program for 1 month after discharge to continue work on time management.

Plan. Discontinue patient from O.T. Recommend attendance at the women's group in outpatient O.T. for 1 month to continue work on time management. Jo Rabson, OTS and Susan Smith, OTR.

Example 4: Cognitive Disabilities

Discharge Summary. August 20, 1985

Data. Patient was referred to O.T. on July 30, 1985, for monitoring of task behavior to assist in titration of medications. Patient was seen in O.T. 12 times. At beginning of treatment, patient's cognitive level was 4, indicating difficulties with attention, new learning, two-step directions, and correction of errors. Goals of O.T. were to provide short-term tasks and assist with problem solving in order to monitor his functional ability and symptoms and to monitor his cognitive level via his task performance as medications were titrated. Methods included basic skills review group and basic crafts. Patient was unable to tolerate the stimulation of other group members when working on craft activity, so he was seen individually for these sessions. At discharge, patient's irritability and paranoid ideation had decreased; however, cognitive level remained at 4.

Interpretation. Cognitive level appears stable at level 4, implying that patient will have a difficult time attending school successfully. The stimulation and cognitive demands of school may precipitate another catastrophic reaction similar to the one preceding this admission. Patient continues to deny limitations in his functioning.

Plan. Discontinue patient from O.T. Recommend structured day program and family counseling to help patient and family adapt to his limitations in functioning. Jo Rabson, OTS and Susan Smith, OTR.

Discharge summaries give a brief synopsis of the patient's O.T. experience. Like the other notes, they should be concise, yet accurate and comprehensive.

*Fig. 4-4. Discharge
summary checklist.*

Check your discharge summaries to see if you have included the following:

Yes   No
____ ____   Date and reason for referral to O.T.
____ ____   Number of O.T. sessions
____ ____   Patient's problems and problem indicators at the beginning of treatment
____ ____   Goals and objectives of O.T. treatment
____ ____   Review of methods used
____ ____   Status of these problems at the patient's discharge or discontinuation of
                  O.T. services
____ ____   Your interpretation of what this information means
____ ____   Recommendations (e.g., home program, contacts with community
                  resources)

Your Turn

Write a discharge summary for the patient you have followed in the past two exercises. Much of the information included in this note will be hypothetic. Nevertheless, every category of information stated in the preceding lists should be included. When done, check your note with the lists in Figs. 4-1 and 4-4 and share the note with a colleague for feedback.

Discharge Summary

Date:

Data:

Interpretation:

Plan:

Signature:

Summary

This section introduced you to the process of writing four types of notes: referral, initial, progress, and discharge. Do not be discouraged if, at first, writing notes takes you longer than you think it should. You will have to write all your notes at least twice (once for your supervisor and then in the chart) for a while. Nevertheless, with feedback and practice, you will become more proficient.

Experience is the name everyone gives to their mistakes.
Oscar Wilde
Lady Windermere's Fan

This chapter introduced you to the process of writing four types of notes: referral, initial, progress, and discharge. All that is left is for you to try it with a patient. It is presumed that in the last two chapters you collected a data base and planned treatment for a patient. Using the guidelines suggested below, organize your data and write an initial note. Pay particular attention to any question or problem you have as you write this note, as it may indicate an area that needs more work. Share your notes with a fellow student or colleague; the shared feedback will help you both develop better note-writing skills.

Initial Note

Category	*Information included*
Data	Results of screening interviews and performance assessment; observations of patient during screening or evaluation; additional evaluations used (title, numeric score [if any], what score means)
Interpretation	Problems and problem indicators; strengths
Plan	Goals; objectives; methods (activity and format)

Initial Note

Date:

Data:

Interpretation:

Plan:

Signature:

Check your note against the following:

Yes	No	Format:
____	____	Are all the important data included?
____	____	Is the note as concise as I can make it?
____	____	Are the grammar and spelling accurate?
____	____	Did I refer to myself in the third person?
____	____	Is it legible?
____	____	Is it dated?
____	____	Is it signed?
____	____	Are the errors corrected accurately?

Have you included the following?

Yes	No	
____	____	Referral data (if no referral note was written)
____	____	Date and type of evaluation(s) given
____	____	Results of interview, evaluations
____	____	What these results mean
____	____	Observations of patient during screening and evaluation
____	____	Patient's problems and problem indicators
____	____	Patient's strengths
____	____	Goals and objectives
____	____	Methods (activities, format)
____	____	Additional information needed (e.g., follow-up evaluation, delay in working on some problems)
____	____	O.T. schedule including date of reassessment

Notes to myself:

Progress Note

If you are able to work with your patient over time, continue this exercise and complete a progress note and discharge summary. If you assessed the patient, but did not provide any of the treatment, then skip it for now. You can review this exercise when you have the opportunity to work with a patient from the beginning to the end of his treatment.

Category	Information included
Data	Patient's attendance at O.T.; O.T. treatment given; reevaluation of patient's status, names of instruments used, numeric score [if any], what score means; observations of patient; relevant patient comments
Interpretation	Changes in patient status from initial evaluation to present; therapist's opinion about the meaning of the data collected so far
Plan	Plan for O.T. treatment (continue previous plan, add new components, delete old components)

Progress Note

Date:

Data:

Interpretation:

Plan:

Signature:

Check your note against the following:

Yes	No	Format:
____	____	Are all the important data included?
____	____	Is the note as concise as I can make it?
____	____	Are the grammar and spelling accurate?
____	____	Did I refer to myself in the third person?
____	____	Is it legible?
____	____	Is it dated?
____	____	Is it signed?
____	____	Are the errors corrected accurately?

Have you included the following?

Yes	No	
____	____	Patient attendance at O.T.
____	____	O.T. treatment given
____	____	Results of further evaluation or re-evaluation
____	____	Relevant observations of patient during O.T.
____	____	Changes in patient status
____	____	Your interpretation of what this information means
____	____	Plan for treatment (additions, deletions, remain the same)

Notes to myself:

Discharge Summary

Finally, write a discharge summary using the information included below:

Category	Information included
Data	Introductory data (date of referral to O.T., reason for referral, number of times seen in O.T.); patient's status at beginning of treatment (specific problems and problem indicators); goals of O.T. treatment; types of methods used; patient's status at discharge, including progress on specific problems noted at beginning of treatment
Interpretation	Therapist's opinion about what above data mean
Plan	Additional recommendations (e.g., home program, community contacts)

Discharge Summary

Date:

Data:

Interpretation:

Plan:

Signature:

Check your note against the following:

Yes *No* Format:
____ ____ Are all the important data included?
____ ____ Is the note as concise as I can make it?
____ ____ Are the grammar and spelling accurate?
____ ____ Did I refer to myself in the third person?
____ ____ Is it legible?
____ ____ Is it dated?
____ ____ Is it signed?
____ ____ Are the errors corrected accurately?

Have you included the following?

Yes *No*
____ ____ Date and reason for referral to O.T.
____ ____ Number of O.T. sessions
____ ____ Patient's problems and problem indicators at the beginning treatment
____ ____ Goals and objectives of O.T. treatment
____ ____ Review of methods used
____ ____ Status of these problems at the patient's discharge or discontinuation of O.T. services
____ ____ Your interpretation of what this information means
____ ____ Recommendations (e.g., home program, contacts with community resources)

Notes to myself:

Summary

This bridge will only take you halfway there
To those mysterious lands you long to see:
Through gypsy camps and swirling Arab fairs
And moonlit woods where unicorns run free.
So come and walk awhile with me and share
The twisting trails and wondrous worlds I've known.
But this bridge will only take you halfway there.
The last few steps you'll have to take alone.

Shel Silverstein
"This Bridge"*

This book introduced you to four basic skills you need to practice psychiatric O.T.: communication, assessment, treatment planning, and documentation. These skills are not unique to psychiatry; they will serve you well in all aspects of O.T. practice. If you have completed the exercises along the way, you will be feeling more confident of your skills and also have some ideas of areas that need more work. As you have learned, you are ultimately responsible for your continued clinical growth. Self-directed learning, or learning you initiate to meet your needs, along with continued self-evaluation are the two most effective methods of developing clinical expertise.

Your final assignment is to take stock of your skills and identify those areas that you feel are strengths and those areas that need continued attention. Look back over the "Your Turn" and "Trying It Out" exercises for specific reminders. Once identified, these areas can be translated into goals for your fieldwork. (You know how to write goals.) Taking stock of your skills at this point will both boost your confidence (you do indeed know how to do some things) and ensure your continued clinical growth (specific goals lead to specific results).

	Strengths	*Areas for improvement*
Communication:		
Assessment:		
Treatment planning:		
Documentation:		

*From *A Light in the Attic: Poems and Drawings* by Shel Silverstein (copyright © 1981 by Snake Eye Music, Inc.; reprinted by permission of Harper & Row, Publishers, Inc.).

My plan for change:

Index

ACL. *See* Allen Cognitive Level Test
Actions, attending, 7–11
Activity
  defined, 130
  format selection in, 140–145
  purposeful, 128–129
  selection of
    background issues in, 128–129
    guidelines for, 130–133
  use of
    structure selection in, 133–136
    teaching methods and, 136–139
Activity Configuration Questionnaire, 77
Administration protocol, for evaluation
    instrument, 64–65
Adolescent Role Assessment, 73
Allen Cognitive Level Test, 59, 81
American Occupational Therapy
    Association
  purposeful activities and, 128
  Uniform Evaluation Checklist, 44
Analogue observation, 79
Anchored rating scales, 76, 78
AOTA. *See* American Occupational
    Therapy Association
Approach, variety in, 152
ARA. *See* Adolescent Role Assessment
Assessment
  evaluation instrument in, 64–87. *See also*
    Evaluation
  practice scheme for, 99–104
  role of theory in, 44–50
  screening process in, 51–63
  terminology of, 42–43
  treatment process and, 42
Atmosphere, of treatment setting, 7
Attending actions, 7–11
Audiovisual aids, as teaching method, 137
Awareness, expansion of, 10

B. H. Battery, the, 83
Back channels, 9–10
Bay Area Functional Performance Evalua-
    tions (BAFPE), 59, 80
Behavior ratings, 78–79
  psychometric properties of, 70
  scales for, 80
Behavioral goals. *See* Outcome goals
Bias, of therapist, 96–97
Blockage, to effective listening, 12–13
  distortions in, 13
Body
  movement of, as teaching method, 137
  position of, 8

Change, self-attribution of, 150–151
Chart review
  case example, 60–62
  in data base establishment, 53–55
  information organization in, 54
  preliminary data synthesis and, 60
Checklists
  of assessment, 76, 77–78
  for notewriting
    discharge summaries, 178
    initial, 173
    of progress, 176
  for referrals, 52

Clarity, of problem, 92
Closed questions, 21
Cognitive disabilities, 47
  activity selection guidelines and, 132
  discharge summary and, 177
  format selection and, 144
  initial note and, 171
  interview content for, 57–58
  performance measure of, 59
  problems, indicators and strengths in,
    90–91
  progress note and, 174
  structure selection and, 135–136
  teaching method selection and, 139
  treatment and, 113–114
Cognitive Level Test
  Allen, 59, 81
  Lower, 59
Collage, the, 83
Comfort, of patient, 10
Common sense responses, 3–4
Communication
  nonverbal. *See* Nonverbal
    communication
  professional behavior and, 2–3
  self-consciousness and, 2
Compensatory model, 151–152
Comprehensive Occupational Therapy
    Evaluation, 59, 80
Concurrent validity, 68
Conditions
  as objective component, 122
  as outcome goal component, 120–121
Congruence, listening and, 14
Construct validity, 68–69
Content
  in group activity, 142
  of message, 6
  validity of, 67–68
COTE. *See* Comprehensive Occupational
    Therapy Evaluation
Criterion
  as objective component, 122
  as outcome goal component, 120
  validity of, 68

Data. *See also* Data base
  collection over time, treatment and, 155
  norms in evaluation of, 65
Data base
  establishment of, case example for,
    60–63
  in screening process, 53–63
"Dead man's error," 120
Demonstration, as teaching method, 136
Diagnosis, in data base establishment,
    53–54
Directed questions, 24
Disability, cognitive. *See* Cognitive
    disabilities
Discharge summaries, 175–178
  checklist for, 178
  practice scheme for, 182–183
Discovery, as teaching method, 136
Documentation, notewriting as. *See* Notes
Double questions, 24
Dysfunction, psychiatric, treatment
    theory for, 112–115

Enlightenment model, 151–152
Environment, treatment setting and, 7
Error
  "Dead man's," 120
  in notes, 167
  in problem identification, 96–98
Evaluation, 64
  instruments, 72–83
    psychometric properties of, 70
    selection of, 83–87
  and principles of measurement, 64–72
  of treatment outcome, 153–155
Expectation, positive, 150
Exploration, as teaching method, 136
Eye contact, 8–9

Face validity, 67
"False positives," 66
Feedback, 26–27
  observation versus interpretation in,
    29–30
  owning message in, 28–29
  positives in, 27–28
Feelings
  categories of, 18
  nonverbal communication of, 14
  paraphrasing and, 18–19
Field trips, as teaching method, 137
Format, for activity, 140–145
Frame of reference, in data base
  establishment, 55–56
Functional performance, 46
  activity selection guidelines and, 131
  discharge summary and, 176
  format selection and, 143
  initial note and, 169
  interview content for, 57
  performance measure of, 58–59
  problems, indicators and strengths in,
    88–89
  progress note and, 173–174
  structure selection and, 134
  teaching method selection and, 138
  treatment and, 112

"Giving feedback," 27
Goals
  outcome. *See* Outcome goals
  service, 126–127
Group Therapy, 140–147
Groups
  activity versus verbal, 140–141
  developmental, 142
  effective use of, 144–145
  versus individual patient treatment, 140
  instrumental, 143
  new, establishment of, 145
    protocol for, 146
  subject content in, 142
  task-oriented, 142
  thematic, 143

Helping, models of, 151–152
"Hey, Dad!" test, 116–117
History of present illness, in data base
  establishment, 55
Hygiene, of patient, 10

IC. *See* Interest Checklist
Initial notes, 168–172
  checklist for, 173
  practice scheme for, 179–180
Instruments, of evaluation, 72–83
  category identification in, 84
  psychometric properties of, 70
  selection of, 83–87
    guide for, 84
Integration, sensory. *See* Sensory
    integration
Interest, in patient, 10
Interest Checklist, 77
Interobserver reliability, 66
Interpretation versus observation, 29–30
Interview. *See also* Listening
  as evaluation instrument, 72, 73
  in data base establishment, 56–58
  Occupational Role History. *See*
    Occupational Role History Interview
  psychometric properties of, 70
  structure of, 33
  tape-recorded. *See* Tape-recorded
    interview

Judgements, listening and, 12

Kohlman Evaluation of Living Skills
  (KELS), 59, 81

LAP. *See* Life Attitude Profile
LCL. *See* Lower Cognitive Level Test
Legal protection, notes and, 167
Leisure Satisfaction Index, 78
Life Attitude Profile, 78
Listening. *See also* Interview
  effective, blockage to, 12–13
    distortions in, 13
  with eyes, 14
  improvement of, 14–15
  levels of, 14–15
Lower Cognitive Level Test, 59
LSI. *See* Leisure Satisfaction Index

Meaning, paraphrasing and, 17–18
Measurement
  error in, 96
  principles of, 64–72
Measures, of outcome, 154–155
Medical model, 151–152
Medications, in data base establishment,
  54–55
Mental status examination, in data base
  establishment, 55
Message
  content of, 6
  and listening with eyes, 14
  nonverbal, 5–6
  ownership, in feedback, 28–29
Midline, outcome goals and, 120–121
Mind set, listening and, 13
Model of human occupation, 46–47
  activity selection guidelines and, 132
  discharge summary and, 177
  format selection and, 144
  initial note and, 170
  interview content for, 57
  performance measure of, 59

Model of human occupation—*Continued*
    problems, indicators and strengths in,
        90
    progress note and, 174
    structure selection and, 135
    teaching method selection and, 138–139
    treatment and, 113
Modeling, 150
Model(s)
    of helping, 151–152
    of human occupation. *See* Model of
        human occupation
Monitoring, participant, 79
Moral model, 151–152

Naturalistic observation, 78–79
Neuropsychologic instruments, 81–82
    examples of, 82
    psychometric properties of, 70
Nonverbal communication, 5–7
    of feelings, 14
Norms, in data evaluation, 65
Notes
    checklist for, 167
    discharge summaries as, 175–178
        checklist for, 178
        practice scheme for, 182–183
    initial, 168–172
        checklist for, 173
        practice scheme for, 179–180
    major functions of, 166
    of progress, 173–175
        checklist for, 176
        practice scheme for, 181–182
    of referral, 167–168
    rules for, 166–167
Nurturing, 10–11

Objectives
    defined, 121–122
    specificity of, 122
Observation
    analogue, 79
    effective listening and, 14
    versus interpretation, 29–30
    naturalistic, 78–79
    of problem, 92
OCA. *See* Occupational Case Analysis
Occupation, human, model of. *See* Model
    of human occupation
Occupational Case Analysis, 73
Occupational Functioning Tool, 73
Occupational Role History Interview,
        34–35, 73
    administration of, 35–36
    interpretation of, 36–38
    self-evaluation, 38
Occupational therapy, domain of concern
    in, 44–50
OFT. *See* Occupational Functioning Tool
Open questions, 20–21
ORHI. *See* Occupational Role History
    Interview
Outcome, of treatment, evaluation of,
        153–155
Outcome goals
    components of, 120–121

defined, 116
    issues affecting setting of, 123–126
Outcomes
    problems and, 118–119
    service type, 126–127
    specificity versus "the fuzzies" in,
        116–117

Paraphrasing, 17
    levels of, 17–20
PARP. *See* Prevocational Assessment of
    Rehabilitation Potential
Participant monitoring, 79
Patient
    preparation of, 5–7
    role in setting of outcome goals, 125–126
    and self-attribution of change, 150–151
Perception, patient's, 150–151
Perceptual defense, listening and, 13
Performance
    as objective component, 122
    as outcome goal component, 120
    demonstration and, as teaching method,
        136
    functional. *See* Functional performance
    measure of, in data base establishment,
        58–59
Person Symbol, 82
Positioning, of body, 7
Positive expectation, 150
Positives
    "false," 66
    in feedback, 27–28
"Practice effect," 66
Precautions, in data base establishment, 55
Predictive validity, 68
Preparation
    of patient, 5–7
    of treatment setting, 7
Prevocational Assessment of Rehabili-
        tation Potential, 80
Primary questions, 22
Prioritization, in problem identification,
        93-94
Problem solving, as teaching method, 137
Problems
    identification of, 88–91
        error sources in, 96–98
        prioritization in, 93–94
        specificity in, 91–93
    and outcome goals, 118–119
    presenting, in data base establishment,
        54
Process goals, 126–127
Professionalism, 2–3
Progress notes, 173–175
    checklist for, 176
    practice scheme for, 181–182
Projective instruments, 82–83
    examples of, 83
    psychometric properties of, 70
Projects, as teaching method, 137
Protocol
    for evaluation instrument
        administration, 64–65
        scoring, 65–67
    for new group establishment, 146
PS. *See* Person Symbol

Psychology, occupational therapy and, 45
Purposeful activity. *See* Activity,
    purposeful

Questionnaires, 76, 77
Questions
    closed, 21
    directed, 24
    double, 24
    format of, 20–21
    open, 20–21
    in ORHI, 35–36
    primary and secondary, 22–23
    why, 25

RAPS. *See* Role Activity Performance Scale
Rating scales
    anchored, 76, 78
    of behavior, 80
RC. *See* Role Checklist
Realism, outcome goals and, 123–125
Referrals, 51–53
    checklist for, 52
    notes for, 167–168
Reification, of problem, 92–93
Relationship, self-esteem enhancement
        through, 148–149
Reliability, in data evaluation, 65–67
Resources, availability of, 56
Responses
    feedback and, 26–30
    to feelings, 18–19
    to immediate situation, 17
    to meaning, 17–18
    questions and, 20–26
    to reasons for feelings, 19
    selection of, 30–32
    tangential, 16
    unrelated, 16
Role Activity Performance Scale, 73
Role balance, ORHI interpretation and, 37
Role Checklist, 78
Role play, as teaching method, 137
Role status, ORHI interpretation and,
        36–37
Routine Task History (RTH), 73
Rushing, listening and, 12–13

SBC Adult Psychiatric Sensory Integration
        Evaluation, 82
Scorable Self-Care Evaluation, 59, 80–81
Scoring protocol, for evaluation
        instrument, 65–67
Screening process
    data base establishment in, 53–63
    referrals in, 51–53
SCSIT. *See* Southern California Sensory
        Integration Tests
SDS. *See* Self-directed Search Questionnaire
Secondary questions, 22–23
Self-attribution, of change, 150–151
Self-consciousness, 2
Self-directed Search Questionnaire, 77
Self-esteem, enhancement of, 148–150
Self-evaluation
    following ORHI, 38
    by therapist, 152–153

Self-monitoring instruments, 72–75
    psychometric properties of, 70
Self-report instruments, 74, 76–77
    examples of, 77–78
    psychometric properties of, 70
Sensory integration, 46
    activity selection guidelines and, 131
    discharge summary and, 176–177
    evaluation of, 65, 82
    format selection and, 143–144
    initial note and, 169–170
    interview content for, 57
    performance measure of, 59
    problems, indicators and strengths in,
        89
    progress note and, 174
    structure selection and, 134–135
    teaching method selection and, 138
    treatment and, 112–113
Sensory overload, listening and, 13
Sequencing, in structuring of activities,
        134
Service goals, 126–127
SIS. *See* Social Interaction Scale
Social chit-chat, 16
Social Interaction Scale, 80
Solutions, listening and, 12
Southern California Sensory Integration
        Tests, 65
Specificity
    of objectives, 122
    in outcome goals, 116–117
    in problem identification, 91–93
SSCE. *See* Scorable Self-Care Evaluation
Strengths, identification of, 95
Structure, in activity, 133–136
Success, defined, 154

Tape-recorded interview, 33–34
    considerations for, 34
    release form for, 34
Task
    evaluations, 79, 81
        examples of, 80–81
        psychometric properties of, 70
    self-esteem enhancement through,
        149–150
    written, as teaching method, 137
Task-Oriented Assessment, 80
Teaching methods, for activity, 136–139
Test-retest reliability, 66
Therapist
    bias of, 96–97
    self-evaluation by, 152–153
    service goals for, 126–127
    varied approach by, 152
Therapy
    association. *See* American Occupational
        Therapy Association
    group. *See* Group therapy
    occupational, domain of concern in,
        44–50
Thinking, listening and, 12–13
Time
    data collection and, 155
    outcome goals and, 123–125
TOA. *See* Task-Oriented Assessment
Tone of voice, 14

Treatment
  activity selection for, 128–133
  activity usage in, 133–147
  evaluating outcome of, 153–159
  expected length of, 55–56
  implementation of, 148–153
  objectives in, 110, 121–123
  outcome goals in, 110, 116–121
    issues affecting setting of, 123–126
    service type, 126–127
  practice scheme for, 156–160
  process for, 42
  role of theory and, 112–115
  setting preparation for, 7

Validity, 67
  construct, 68–69
  content, 67–68
  criterion, 68
  face, 67
Value judgements, feedback and, 26–27
Voice, tone of, 14

Why questions, 24
World view, development of, 151–152
Written tasks, as teaching method, 137